Holey Ship High in Transport

I Had Cancer

BY MATTHEW G. WALTON D.O. AND GARY A. WALTON

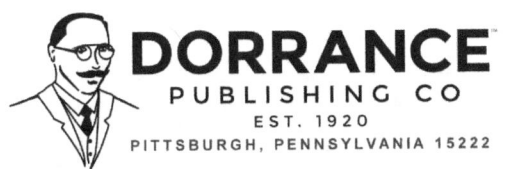

DORRANCE
PUBLISHING CO
EST. 1920
PITTSBURGH, PENNSYLVANIA 15222

Dorrance Publishing Co
701 Smithfield Street
Pittsburgh, PA 15222
Visit our website at *www.dorrancebookstore.com*

ISBN: 978-1-4809- 1254-0
eISBN: 978-1-4809-1576-3

Dedication

To Mom and Dad, who never left my side.

Preface

First thing first: *Why am I writing this?* This is a hard question to answer. The reason it is a hard question is because it implies purpose, and as you will see later, purpose is everything—well, almost. I guess the most basic reason I had for writing this was the simple fact that I had a story to tell. Who heard the story was not important at first. What was important was the simple fact that I got to tell it, but why did I have to tell it? For too long I would just rehearse single individual events in my mind. Never had I tried to piece together all the individual fragments to see what they would form. In other words, what I really needed to do was to take everything I experienced from this specific time in my life and try to piece it all together to understand what it all meant. The following pages all started out with this idea, with me just trying to organize my experiences and thoughts concerning a major event in my life.

In the beginning this writing served as therapy, a type of psychoanalysis if you will. In reading this in some sense you can think of yourself as my shrink. As you read you can just imagine me lying on the couch next to you. Please also imagine that this takes place in a free clinic as you will not be paid to listen to me ramble.

I know that I said who I told this story to was not important, but that was in the beginning. Then I had an idea. Maybe my story could potentially benefit someone else—perhaps someone who was having a similar experience, but then again anyone who experiences cancer has their own unique experience. To say that reading my experience can help you with yours would be condescending, so I canned that idea. My next thought was that maybe I could use my experience for somebody who wanted to be entertained, as a way to make them laugh, but then again my sense of humor could be perceived as a little twisted and maybe quite different from yours, so I canned that idea too. I don't want to offend anyone. Maybe these pages are for someone who knew someone else who had cancer. Maybe this will help them to understand what someone else is going through, but I come back full circle and will say it again: Anyone who experiences cancer has their own unique experience. Listening to my story will only place you in my shoes and no one else's.

So again, why am I telling this story? Why am I spending countless hours at night dictating these pages? Well, I know that I am writing this for someone, for some particular reason, although I am not quite certain for whom and what that reason is, but there is someone out there who will get something out of this. For this reason I present my story. Make sense? I sure hope so. I am getting tired of answering my own questions.

Part I: Why Me?
The Prequel

Every good story nowadays seems to need a prequel, so let me start by saying I never thought I would be in the hospital again. Yes, I said again. Having one traumatic life-altering event as a child is rare enough, but having two has to be a violation of some statistical law of averages. So let's get started.

It was August of 1988. I was five and our family had just returned home from vacation, and I mean we'd *just* gotten home. The van was in the driveway and was not even unpacked yet. Our neighbors across the street were holding our mail and my dad crossed the street to pick it up, and I, for some reason, had to tag along. It is the return home where things start to get blurry, but don't worry, our neighbors were having a party and many of them would be witnesses to the upcoming event. I remember stepping onto the street. The important thing to remember here is that I am still walking, because after the next second I will not take another step for four months. The last thing I recall as I stepped onto the street is everything fading to black and my dad yelling my name. Unbeknownst to me, a fifteen-year-old was taking his dad's motorcycle out for a joy ride. Apparently this young man's joy ride came into contact with little old me. I was told that the kid on the motorcycle broke his arm. On the other hand, according to all the partying bystanders, I took a trip through the air. I was sent flying that day and landed back on the pavement about sixty feet from where I once stood.

The next memory I have is in the emergency room of the local hospital. I remember being surrounded by a bunch of people I didn't know and they were wearing masks so I could not identify them. To set the mood, think of it like an alien abduction, waking up and being surrounded by unknown figures. I remember screaming my mom's name. I remember being told to go back to sleep. After that things get fuzzy again. Apparently yours truly got to go flying a second time that day. This time it was in a helicopter. I was flown to Children's Hospital of Pittsburgh, and this would be my first of two major events requiring that hospital's assistance. I broke some bones in my legs. I broke some bones in my arms and I fractured a few ribs. Wait, there's more: I injured my liver too.

I was fitted into a body cast and I remained entombed for a total of three months. The first cast I was in was made of plaster and I remember it being very hot because of one particular incident. Either the power or the air conditioner failed, because the memory I have engraved into my head is my mom pleading with someone on the phone to get things working again due to the fact that her son (that's me) was about to have a heat stroke.

Let me now address that question lingering in the back of your mind. It is the same question I am always asked when I tell someone I was in a body cast. The question: "How do you use the bathroom in a body cast?" The answer: "I basically had two strategically placed holes, a big plastic pan, a urine bottle, and a very devoted mom." It wasn't very glamorous, but neither was the rest of my life during those three months. I basically served as furniture. Let's face it, I wasn't going anywhere. After a few weeks things improved, but only slightly. I did teach myself how to scoot around on the carpet due to the fact that one arm and one leg was not completely casted, and speaking of teaching, my first half of kindergarten was spent homebound. The kindergarten teacher actually came to the house. This was also the first time I was taught homebound, implying that there will likely be a second.

After two different casts and three months, I was finally freed from my tomb. Thankfully, the liver healed on its own. Now, when you don't use your muscles for three months, don't expect to walk right off the bat. In fact, your first lesson is just trying to move your extremities. Not moving for three months causes your muscles to atrophy and tighten up. Thus step one was stretching and step two was learning to roll over. After I mastered this concept, I moved to sitting up. From sitting I progressed to crawling. Once crawling was mastered, I slowly began to learn to walk again. I went through all the same steps as an infant and it took a while, but I was walking again. Now you would think by playing the odds that the chances of me having to undergo another major medical event would be low, but if you picked up my foreshadowing earlier you know this is not the case. Lightning can strike the same place twice, and it did for me. It struck me right in the head, figuratively speaking. Eight years after this event I would be going back to Children's Hospital, and why was I going back? I was going back because my twin brother finally decided to show himself. *Say what?*

The Ominous Signs

The word *ominous* is often used in relation to the weather. When a storm approaches we say the sky looks ominous, but knowing what the sky looks like before a storm allows us to come to that conclusion. If we have never seen a storm, before how do we predict what is about to come? There is a parallel between this and the first signs of there being something wrong with me other than the usual. When the first symptoms appeared, everybody was cognizant of them but nobody knew what they meant. Since nobody knew what they meant there was no cause for alarm. Sometimes the signs are only ominous in retrospect.

It was summer again, the summer between my seventh and eighth grade year. My family and I happened to be spending the day at a friend's cabin in the mountains. The first symptom arose that evening as the sun began to set. While strolling the campground, people started commenting on my eyes. The basic comment I got was that my eyes looked funny. I do remember looking in the mirror that evening, and they were right. My eyes did look funny and my pupils were the problem. They were dilated. My only explanation for this rested on the fact that it was dark out and with this explanation I simply brushed any concerns aside. The only problem with this reasoning was that the morning dawn did nothing to correct the problem. Still nobody thought much of it.

Headaches were the second symptom to present. At first they too were of little concern. They started out as your typical, average, everyday headache. They were mild, intermittent, and non-debilitating. Non-debilitating? I never presumed a headache could be debilitating—at least up to this point—but as the next few days came and went, the headaches became the sign that something was definitely wrong. No longer was I running around like before. The pain in my head began to intensify to a point where I almost became incapacitated. I was now bed bound because falling asleep became my only refuge from the pain. I can only describe the pain as a horrible pressure, and oddly enough this will end up being an exact description of the truth. It was around this time that my parents started getting very concerned as well. I was no longer myself. Well, I was still me, but I was not acting like me and I think that is what scared them. The next thing I knew I had an appointment with the pediatrician.

It had been about a week since the cabin in the mountains. During this timeframe, at no point did I suspect what was really going on. At no point did I figure my twin was finally going to make his presence known.

The Explanation

I do not recall much of what happened at the pediatrician's office, but I do remember a definite change in mood as the examination progressed. What I knew at this point was that I had big eyes and a really bad headache. I am almost certain that the pediatrician picked up on a few other things as well and all he needed to do was to take a closer look at my eyes. The eyes are a remarkable organ. We can tell so much about a person just by looking at their eyes. The eye is the only window a physician has to look inside the body. Only in the eyes can the physician directly observe structures such as arteries and nerves. Nowhere else in the body can one see these things without the aid of a scalpel. In the back of the eye sits the retinal arteries and the optic nerve. The optic nerve is special because it is also the second cranial nerve. The cranial nerves are special because they are direct extensions of the brain itself. Hence pathology in the brain can sometimes be seen by visualizing the nerve. When the doctor saw my optic nerve I am sure he saw some swelling. Add this to the fact that I had a terrible headache, and now one could deduce that there was pressure building in my brain. Further examination of my eyes would also reveal two other phenomena. The first was that I couldn't look up. I could extend my neck to see objects above me but I couldn't move my eyes up. The second was my argyle pupils. (Before I go any further there may be some medical personal reading this, and to them, let me say that I did not have syphilis. Although everyone equates argyle pupils with syphilis, there are a few rare conditions that can produce the same phenomena. Again, I do not have syphilis.) Argyle pupils are pupils that will not react or constrict to light but will with accommodation. Accommodation is when you look at something very close and your eyes converge inward. In short, my pupils would accommodate but they would not react.

Now my pediatrician was starting to assemble the puzzle pieces. The first piece said that the pressure in this kid's head is building. The second piece said this kid has Parinaud Syndrome. Parinaud Syndrome, or dorsal midbrain syndrome, is actually a collection of symptoms. The first are pupils that accommodate but do not react. The second is the inability to look up. What makes this collection of symptoms so important is that it tells the doctor that there is something pushing on the center of my brain, oh S.H.I.T. (more on the whole S.H.I.T. thing later).

Now we had to see what was going on inside my head. For that I would need a CT scan. From the doctor's office it was a thirty-minute drive to Children's Hospital of Pittsburgh. If I remember correctly, on the drive to the hospital I still was not sure what exactly was going on, but I would soon find out.

I remember very little of the actual CT scan. One thing I do remember was that the scan was not even finished and already the technician was on the phone talking to somebody. There was a look of concern in her eyes. I'd gotten that look now twice that day, and needless to say, I was now worried. The next thing I remember is my dad and I sitting in an exam room. We sat there for some time not really knowing what was going on. I do recall telling my father that I was scared. My dad must've been nervous to because when I told him that there were no words of comfort. The only thing he could say was, "Me too." Eventually a neurosurgeon walked in the room along with a fellow and resident. It was at this point that I found out I had a mass in the center of my brain, a region of the brain known as the pineal region.

All of my symptoms were related to this tumor. As you may or may not know the brain sits in a pool of fluid. This cerebrospinal fluid, or CSF, drains from the front of your head toward the back and down your spine. In regard to the headaches, the tumor served as a dam of sorts, blocking the flow of fluid causing a buildup of pressure. As I said before, pressure was an exact description of the headache. If I would have waited a little bit longer the pressure in my head may have built up to the point where my brain may have herniated out of my skull. That's bad, by the way.

Diagnosis Number One

My neurosurgeon, Dr. Albright, was a brilliant man and you could tell just by talking to him. Any question I asked would cause him to pause and think. You could almost hear the gears turning in his head as he pondered my questions. I imagine he was trying to not just answer the question but to answer the question behind the question while at the same time trying to predict the consequences of his answer. Basically, the man had a great intellect. At some point during our conversations I also learned that this man was either going to be a doctor or a pastor. It seemed like an odd pairing at the time, but you could see the religious side of him. He appeared very pious. When I asked him why he didn't become a pastor, his answer was to the effect that being a doctor also served the needs of him wanting to be a pastor. In the end, I'm glad he chose medicine, for he would be the first of many who were responsible for saving my life.

As I said before, I had many conversations with Dr. Albright, but the first conversation dealt with the question of what exactly was in my head. The answer I got was not the answer I was expecting. It ended up I would need a biopsy. My second question, though asked a little differently at the time, was how in the hell do you biopsy a mass in the center of my brain. The answer to this question was very carefully. The first surgical procedure I had would kill two birds with one stone. Thank God I'm not a bird. The surgeon went through the top of my head and retrieved a sample of the tumor for biopsy while at the same time placing a shunt of some sort which allowed the fluid in my brain to flow properly. Once the shunt was placed my headaches were gone, but the procedure left me with a nice scar. If I were to shave my head today it would appear as if a horse kicked me right on the top of my head.

The biopsy revealed that the tumor was something called a germinoma. I do not recall if it was malignant or benign. What I do remember was that I was being very stubborn at the time. Vacation was coming in about a week and our family has gone on vacation to the same place on the same week since I was born. (If you recall when I was hit by the motorcycle we had just gotten home from vacation. We were planning to go to the exact same place.) After pleading with Dr. Albright and with my parents, our family did go on vacation for five of the planned seven days. Looking back at my actions I can see the stupidity of my request (why would I go out of state if I had a tumor in my head?) but I might have been driven by a higher power, as you will see. A simple inspection of this section's title (Diagnosis Number One) should lead you to the conclusion that the subject material mentioned here is not over.

Diagnosis Number Two

We returned from the beach early as planned and I was right back in the hospital. I was now scheduled to undergo a procedure known as the gamma knife. Although it is called the gamma knife, there is no actual knife. Instead the gamma knife will cut or destroy tissue with energy. It shoots several low-intensity beams of radiation onto a single point inside the body, thereby giving that single point a high dose of radiation. In my case it would be aimed at a point in the center of my brain. You can almost think of it as being like the Death Star, which had the death ray that could destroy planets. All the smaller beams of energy came together to create something more powerful. The only difference between the gamma knife and the Death Star is that with the gamma knife your head is not supposed to explode.

If you're not familiar with the procedure I can honestly say that you will get screwed. The day starts with them faceting this apparatus onto your head. This requires the use of tiny screws that are drilled into your skull to hold the apparatus in place. Then with this big device screwed onto your head, they send you to the MRI to precisely measure the location of the tumor in order to aim the death ray device or gamma knife. The MRI pinpointed the exact location of my tumor, but it also shows that my tumor had doubled in size. This could have only have occurred if I went on vacation, and why is this important? This is not typical of the tumor I was diagnosed with. The Gamma Knife was canceled, and you may think that I got screwed for nothing, but fortunately I did get another surgery out of this and another biopsy was performed. This second biopsy revealed I had a malignant mixed germ cell tumor. First, the word *malignant* means cancer or the ability of tumor cells to migrate to other parts of my body. So what does mixed germ cell mean? Remember before when I mentioned my twin brother showing up? A mixed germ cell tumor is a tumor comprised of all three germ layers, giving it the potential capability to grow entire human tissues and organs. Basically, what I had was a very unorganized person living in my head. There is a remote possibility that this tumor may have been the remnant of a twin that never came to fruition while in utero. Anyway, the treatment plan had completely changed. I would now need to have this tumor surgically removed—and remember, this tumor is still sitting in the center of my brain.

Brain Surgery

Technically, I had already had two minor brain surgeries, but now I was about to have the real thing. Someone was about to remove a large piece of my skull to manipulate brain tissue to then remove foreign tissue from the center of my brain. My recollection of all the events that occurred that day are sketchy, and I'm sure I was nervous, but at the time I was not trying to think about anything, thus resulting in the few memories I have of this event.

The morning of the surgery, I remember having to wake up very early and driving to the hospital while it was still dark. I never saw them, but from what I was told my entire extended family showed up at the hospital as well. I was reported to be in surgery for about eight hours. Dr. Albright did the surgery and was able to remove all visible portions of the tumor. Amazingly, he did this without producing mental damage, but my post-surgical brain mass did end up being less than the pre-surgical. If you look at my postsurgical MRIs you will see some scarring in certain areas of my brain, and if you look close enough you will actually see that a small part of my superior colliculus is missing. This part of my brain was likely damaged by the tumor and had to come out with it. Post-surgery, upon seeing Dr. Albright, my father's first question was, "It didn't go very well, did it?" but what he soon learned was that the doctor was just exhausted. I cannot begin to imagine the amount of patience, concentration, and skill it takes to perform that operation.

The surgery was now over and the scarring on my head was now complete. I told you before about the one on top of my head making it look like I got kicked by a horse, and I now had a scar that ran the entire back of my head, from top to bottom. When I asked the doctor how many stitches I received, thinking I may be able to get in the Guinness Book of World Records, his response was, "I lost count." So much for being in the record books.

Speaking of conversing with the doctor, my mom speaks of an incident that occurred between the surgeon and me during this time. Supposedly, while speaking with the surgeon, I yelled at him because I was having neck pain. The surgeon's response was, "Matt, what do you expect? You just had brain surgery." Apparently in some smart-aleck tone, my response was, "You did brain surgery not neck surgery." It left an impression in my mom's memory, though I have no memory of this event ever taking place. I hate to think of the fact that I might have yelled at a person who was directly involved in saving my life. If it did happen, I blame it on the drugs.

There was also another new scar I began to notice after surgery, only this scar was not on my head. It was on my chest. Not only was there a scar and stitches but there was a large lump there as well (I know what you are thinking, and I was not growing breasts). Now I don't remember ever being informed that I would be getting this device, but while I was under during brain surgery, I had a medi-port placed under my skin a few inches above my right nipple. A medi-port is a device that makes the process of giving IV medications and taking blood a lot simpler and prevents your arms from being torn up with needles. As mentioned, the device sits right under your skin and can be accessed by placing a needle through the skin. The device then has tubing which connects it to a vein that leads directly to your heart. The first time I had it accessed it hurt like hell. Sometime afterward I was told that there was cream to numb the skin. I do recommend it. Once I got my hands on it I never left home without it. I got this medi-port so that it would be easier to get IV medications, but what IV medications would I be getting? Survey says: chemotherapy.

Chemotherapy

It was a few days after brain surgery and I was recuperating in the hospital. I didn't even get to go home. In time I was just transferred to another floor, the Hematology/Oncology floor. The hospital had an entire section dedicated to this specialty. I have to go on a quick tangent here—just bear with me. At the time, I hated the word *chemo*. People used it as a shorthand word for chemotherapy. I didn't like it because I thought something as serious as chemotherapy should not be degraded with some ad-lib nickname. I mean, for God's sake, these drugs could kill me just as easily. I made everyone around me use the word *chemotherapy* and I corrected anyone who used the word *chemo*. Till this day I still remember the name of the chemotherapy drugs. There were three. Their names were bleomycin, VP-16, and carboplatin. I can even recall what the drugs looked like. I remember that the carboplatin came in the largest IV bag while the bleomycin just came in a syringe. I would receive all three of these drugs over a three-day period while in the hospital. There were a total of three sessions and each session was separated by a few weeks.

On my inaugural arrival to the floor, all the rooms were taken but one, which happened to be the bone marrow transplant room. Now all the rooms on this floor were designed to be sterile, but this room took it to the extreme. Patients who routinely used this room had received so much chemotherapy that their body no longer had the ability to fight off disease. This room helped put everything into perspective. Before you walked into the room you had to pass through an airlock of sorts. While in the airlock you had to wash your hands, and the water in the sink was controlled by foot pedals to keep your hands as clean as possible. While walking into the actual room, you had to walk over a mat covered in a sticky substance that removed particles from your shoes. Nothing from the outside got into this room. Once in the room you were isolated from the outside environment. The room had its own atmospheric controls so that the air you breathed in the room was different than that in the hallway outside. I almost expected a person dressed in one of those radiation outfits with an oxygen tank on his back to walk in any second.

I remember the first night I spent in that room, and I remember it quite vividly. One of my parents was in the chair beside me and I didn't sleep much that night. I laid there in the dark and stared at the ceiling. I recall this next event as clear as the day it happened. While staring at the ceiling I whispered, "Please, God, don't let me die." After I said this I thought to myself, *You will never forget this moment*, and I haven't. Another reason I remember this night so well was that it was the first time I had my medi-port accessed.

Starting chemotherapy was also around the time I met Dr. Michael Wollman. Dr. Wollman was a hematology oncologist and he was in charge of my chemotherapy; he eventually became the person in charge of my cancer treatment. This man was probably the most important person involved in saving my life. Dr. Albright saved me in the short term, and it is because of Dr. Wollman that I am here today. I will have a lot more to say about him later, but let's continue with the story.

As mentioned before, I had three sessions of chemotherapy. Each session involved a three-day stay in the hospital. After each stay I would go home, only to return a few days later with a fever. Chemotherapy mostly works by killing cells as they divide, so cells that divide rapidly are most easily killed. Cancer cells usually divide rapidly. That is why they use chemotherapy but there are many cells in your body that also divide rapidly. These cells are mainly found in your blood and would include things such as red and white blood cells. A normal white blood cell count is about 10. After I received chemotherapy my count dropped as low as 0.7, if I remember correctly. In essence I was an AIDS patient without HIV. I was even placed on prophylactic antibiotics during my entire treatment period to prevent opportunistic infections which could cause pneumonia. I use the word *antibiotics* and not *antibiotic* because I was on two different medications. The first medication was Dapsone, but I developed methemoglobin with this drug. What is methemoglobin? It's basically a disorder where your red blood cells have a hard time carrying oxygen. In my case, I literally turned blue. The day I was diagnosed I was wearing a white shirt and red sweatpants and I was the all-American boy, according to Dr. Wollman. Once I was diagnosed as the all-American boy, the Dapsone was stopped and I had to instead receive breathing treatments once a month.

When you're white count gets as low as mine was, you can basically infect yourself with the normal bacteria in places like your intestine, which are supposed to be there to help not hurt. A few days after chemotherapy I would wake up in the middle of the night sweating profusely with a fever. My parents would call the hospital and we would be told to come on down. I would get IV antibiotics prophylactically just in case I caught some horrible bug. They would always use the same antibiotic. I am not kidding when I say this the drug looked like urine. It was yellow. It was bubbly, and it smelled bad. For my fevers I would spend about two days in the hospital until my fever resolved and my white count came up. Eventually I had so much trouble with my white count dropping that I was eventually put on Nupogen. This was a drug designed to stimulate the growth of white blood cells and it wasn't a pill. I had to inject it every day.

My white count was not the only thing that dropped. My red cells would do the same, and again, this was a common side effect. Once I would go home I would have to get my finger pricked every couple days to see where my hemoglobin was. I became a regular at the local lab. Like clockwork, chemotherapy would drop my hemoglobin to the point that I would have to get someone else's blood. People actually donated blood specifically for me. Believe it or not, even my own dentist donated blood. I remember trips to the outpatient cancer center. Walking downhill to the center would make me short of breath. After I received the blood I was able to walk uphill without a problem. With the blood I often had to get platelets too. I actually remember the first time I received platelets. I was in the hospital with a fever. As soon as those platelets entered me I got the worst case of chills you could imagine and my temperature went up to about 104°F. You would not believe the number of nurses that come running when your temperature goes that high in the matter of minutes. After that experience I never got blood or platelets without first being doped up on Benadryl.

By the time chemotherapy was over, I had lost all my hair. I can even recall the day when most of my hair came out. I woke up one morning and noticed a lot of hair on the pillow. I was warned beforehand and I was told that when I combed my hair my hair would just comb right out. Now I was told this day would come, but I was not prepared. On that day I could not comb my hair, knowing what it would do. My dad had to do it for me, and within a few seconds I was bald—well, not quite. I had a few patches of hair left, which made me look more emaciated than anything else. Hence the decision was made to shave the rest.

My dad drove me down to the local hair salon and he went in to speak to the manager. I was escorted into the salon through the back door and the manager there shaved my head in the salon's kitchen away from everybody else. Once I was completely bald I always wore a hat. I could no longer hide the scars on my head. I didn't want to be stared at or have the idea that I was being watched. After my hair left me, for the next few months one of my main concerns was how my hair would come back. One of my biggest fears was my hair would grow back red. This can happen you know. When it did grow back it was slightly darker and a whole lot thinner.

The Spinal Tap

Toward the end of my chemotherapy I had to have this wonderful procedure known as a spinal tap. This procedure would help determine if any cancer cells were still present in my central nervous system. Unlike some previous events, I remember this event quite well. You would too if you had one without any sedation. Everything starts out with me waiting in the procedure room of the outpatient hematology/oncology clinic. I then had the pleasure of meeting the anonymous resident or fellow who was chosen to perform the procedure. I guess everybody has to learn at some point, right? They first have you lie on your side, and then you curl up into a ball. Apparently this helps to open the space between the vertebrae. My dad helped to hold me in this position, which meant that he got to watch. I should mention that this is a man who has a hard time with blood. The fellow numbed the skin in my lower back with lidocaine. She then palpated for the soft disc between two of my lumbar vertebrae and attempted to place a five- to six-inch needle into my back. She was at this for some time and my dad was getting queasy. What I felt was not really a sharp pain but more of a dull pressure. This dull pressure persisted for some time due to the fact that the fellow was now on her sixth attempt. Thankfully the nurse got the attending physician who was able to finish the job. When this was all over, Dad had to sit down. He may have suffered more than I did. In the end we had about five small test tubes filled with a clear fluid that came directly from my spinal canal.

Upon analysis, the fluid was free of any tumor cells and I never had to have a spinal tap again. Now I was onto the next stage of treatment. This phase did not consist of drugs and there was no surgery. In fact I could not even see what they were about to apply and neither could those who were applying it. The treatment I was about to receive was that of pure energy. This energy, if not harnessed properly, could in turn create another cancer. Now was the time for radiation.

Radiation

Beginning radiation therapy was a time of change. Of all the changes, the most significant was no more nights in the hospital. From now on things were done on an outpatient basis, but this did not mean I would be away from the hospital. Nights were spent in my own bed, but days were still spent at Children's. For the next couple months I would be driven to and from the hospital every day Monday through Friday. The drive to the hospital was about an hour. My treatment at the hospital was about an hour, and again the drive home was another hour. My parents did most of the driving. Every now and then a neighbor would pitch in and offer to drive me down. Life during radiation soon became very monotonous and repetitive. Wait, didn't I say this was a time of change?

Before starting radiation therapy, they had to precisely measure where to shoot it. What they wanted to do was make small tattoo marks on my head and spine. I absolutely refused this. I think it was the idea of having a permanent reminder of what I was about to go through that turned me away from the tattooing. So instead of a few tiny tattoo marks they took magic markers and turned my head and back into a tic-tac-toe board. They also made me a mask. This mask was actually a mold of my face. When I would lay on the table to receive the radiation this mask would be placed over my face so that I could not move my head. Till this day my mask sits in the back of my closet.

A standard day of radiation went like this. Upon arriving I would sign in and sit in the waiting room until they called my name. When I was called the nurse would escort me back to the treatment room. The room was like a giant bank safe. I would walk in through the vault door, lay down on the table, and my head would rest on a large foam triangle. I then would have my custom-fitted mask placed over my face. Laser beams from the machine where then aimed to all the corresponding points drawn on my head. At this point the tech would leave the room and close the vault door. The whole time I was monitored with video cameras. I always knew when the radiation beam was turned on. I basically heard a loud humming sound, but believe it or not, I could also smell when the radiation was on. I didn't actually smell the radiation but the ozone created by the radiation.

The treatment had one minor side effect. The radiation to my spine would upset my stomach, causing me to vomit a few times. Most of the time I could make it to the toilet, though there was this one time when my mom and I were still in the car driving home, and when you have to hurl you have to hurl. It was everywhere. Sorry, Mom.

Post Treatment

There was no sign of any cancer once treatment was over (thank God) but there were new problems (oh S.H.I.T.). The first problem was a hormone problem.

Several months after treatment was over, I was diagnosed with severe growth hormone deficiency. Simply stated, my body no longer produces growth hormone. This problem did not stem from the tumor; instead, it stemmed from the radiation treatment. The radiation may have killed cancer cells, but it also played a number on my pituitary gland.

I can remember the day the doctor told me about my diagnosis. I literally broke down in tears due to the fact that I had another problem to deal face. At the time it felt like I would never get away from this illness. It was as if this process would never end.

If I had never received radiation treatment, I would now likely have a normal pituitary gland and I may have been a few inches taller, but it would have only been for a short time due to the fact that I would now be dead. Being that I enjoy life, I must live with the fact that my body no longer produces the hormone. The consequence is that I now have to inject it every night. It is very similar to an insulin injection. I use a pen-like device and inject the medicine subcutaneously into either my stomach or my leg. I know your next question. If I'm no longer going to grow anymore, why take the growth hormone? This is how it was explained to me: I need to keep my levels within a certain range to prevent certain conditions over the long term such as heart problems which are known to occur in people with chronically low growth hormone levels. I assure you I am not taking it to grow stronger or to compete in the Tour de France.

Once the cancer was gone, the problems with my eyes still persisted. I still had parinaud syndrome and the double vision. The parinaud syndrome is permanent and I will have to spend the rest of my life with my abnormal pupils and my inability to look up. I will never get that missing piece of my superior colliculus back. One thing that could potentially be fixed was my double vision. This was due to an eye muscle problem, caused by the tumor, causing my left eye to deviate laterally. The best way to describe how I saw at that time is as follows. Imagine driving down the road and seeing the cars in front of you moving in the same direction as you but also having cars in the opposite lane coming right at you as well.

As mentioned, this problem could be fixed but I would again need surgery. This time it was eye muscle surgery. An eye muscle was actually disconnected from the eyeball and repositioned. The first time I had the surgery it didn't work, but I was told this may happen. Nonetheless I was getting a little frustrated. The second time I had surgery the problem was corrected by about 90 percent, which means most of the time I don't see double but if my eyes get tired I will look at you and you will have four eyes, literally. To help with this I now wear glasses with a prism that adjust my vision in such a way so I do not have a problem about 99 percent of the time.

I have a unique memory from the second eye surgery. I'm not sure what they put me on to knock me out, but toward the end of the surgery I remember waking up while still on the surgical table when they called out my name. All that I remember seeing was a bright white light. I know what you're thinking, but this light was from a surgical lamp. I assure you I didn't die on the table. Upon waking I remember the doctors asking me to move my eyes in different directions, and once they stop talking to me everything went blank again. The next thing I knew I was in the recovery room.

After treatment I also started to have a lot of problems with anxiety as well. It probably started with just worrying about whether or not the cancer would come back. I was very vigilant in trying to prevent this, and I think this also produced a lot of anxiety for me later, as I will explain. Throughout the cancer treatment process, I always did what I needed to do that exact moment to prevent problems further down the line. I was always at the doctor's office on time. I never missed an appointment. I never missed lab draws. I always took the prescribed medications. I never missed a radiation treatment. Eventually I think this idea started to take hold in everyday life. I would always try to get things done as soon as possible, and if left to sit my thoughts would dwell on that until it was completed. This produced a lot of unwanted anxiety.

It took some time—several years—but I began to understand that the way we think influences the way we feel. Even today I have to remain conscious of the thoughts that sit in the back of my head and how they are influencing my day-to-day life.

The End

As mentioned, I spent my entire eighth-grade year in treatment and I was taught homebound during this entire period. I returned to school the following year. For a few years I had to follow-up with an MRI every few months. When all these MRIs of my head were normal, future scans became more spread out to the point that I was being scanned once a year. Even these routine scans were eventful at times. I distinctly remember one incident. With each MRI I would receive contrast dye in an IV. During one visit they used a different brand or formulation of contrast and it made me sick. What made the problem worse was that I had just eaten lunch, and when my parents took me for these visits we usually had a nice big lunch. That nice big lunch was all over the hospital's expensive MRI. Once it was ten years post-treatment, the scans were finally stopped.

Part 2:
HOLEY S.H.I.T I HAD CANCER
It's All Relative

My first thought after being told I had cancer was *Why me?* but there was one event that put things into perspective. This story takes place while I was in the hospital. I was in the hospital because I had a fever and since I had a fever I needed IV urine. My roommate during this visit was a young male child. This toddler, like the rest of us on the floor, was a cancer patient. His lungs, though, were in perfect working order, I assure you. He cried all night. It had to be some kind of record, and consequently I did not sleep. I will admit that I was pissed in the morning and about to cry myself. The child's mom was there trying to comfort him, but her efforts were in vain.

At some point the next day my dad began to converse with the mom of the amazing crying baby. This woman was always wearing a hat, and at first I thought nothing of it. That was until she removed it. When she did this it came to my attention that she was bald. I assure you this was not a Sinead O'Connor fan or the most recent fashion trend at the time. She had the stigmata of every other patient on the floor. Eventually she admitted to my father that she was a cancer patient too. What type of cancer she had I cannot recall for certain, but it may have been breast cancer.

My mom till this day will not talk about my cancer treatment because it is just too hard for her. Now imagine this mother. She knew exactly what her child was going through, and I could not begin to imagine the empathy she felt for her son and the pain that must have come with that. Whenever I felt sorry for myself, I would think of this night in the hospital. When you think you're the only one who was dealt a bad hand, remember there is always someone worse off than you. Learn humility.

"Humility is the foundation of all the other virtues hence, in the soul in which this virtue does not exist there cannot be any other virtue except in mere appearance."

-Saint Augustine

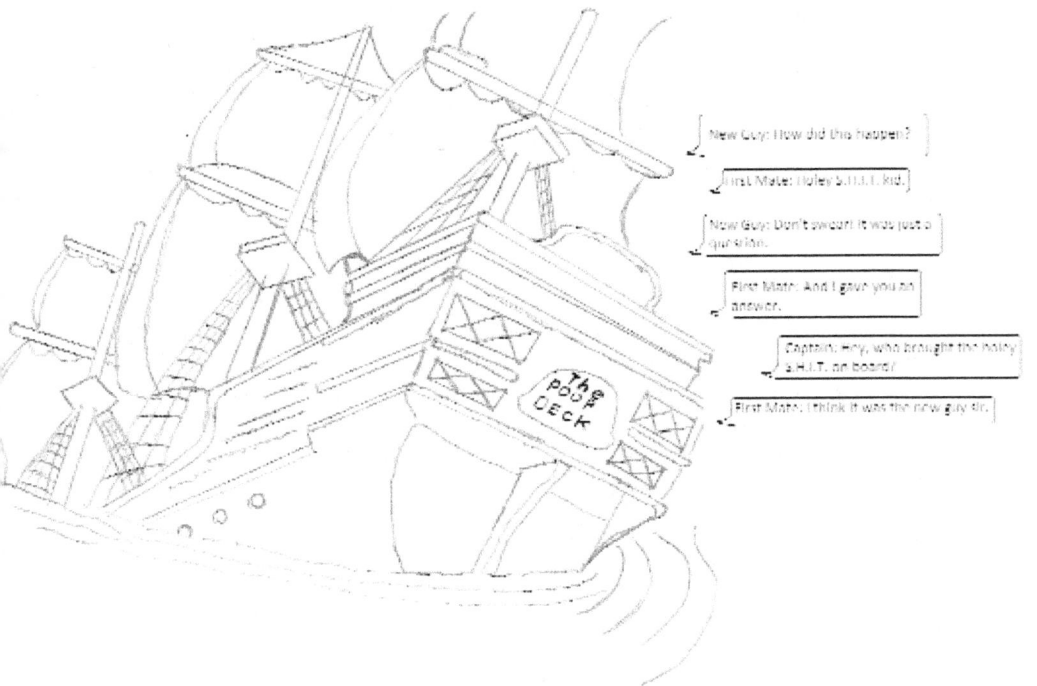

An Explanation on Humor

How we remember something can influence how we feel, and recalling an event concerning cancer has the potential to be a depressing event for all people involved. In lieu of this, one needs to decide how to frame his or her past experiences when those experiences have the potential to become very upsetting. People do this in different ways. For example, my mother just doesn't think about it. When I think about my past experience with cancer, most of the time it is about the positives and often those positives were the events that made me laugh. I would like to explain how some doctors initially used this concept with me. As you recall, one of my presenting symptoms were my eyes. My pupils would not react to light but would shrink with accommodation. In essence they would accommodate but not react. It is the phrase, *accommodate but not react,* that doctors use as a punch line. I am not making this up. Two different distinguished doctors told me the same thing. My world renowned neurosurgeon gave me the diagnosis of whore's eyes, while my ophthalmologist said I had prostitute pupils. Get it? I hope so because I am not explaining this one.

You may have noticed the title Holey S.H.I.T. I Had Cancer. This too is an attempt to reframe a concept with humor. First off *shit* is not a word commonly used in my vocabulary, perhaps due to its vulgarity, but the word Holey S.H.I.T. is acceptable. The reason why is because I have reframed the concept or meaning of the phrase. When someone asks me why I'm using such language, I tell them the following.

Years ago, before the advent of food preservation, many had to grow their own food. To ensure a good quality crop, people were dependent upon a good fertilizer. Before the advent of artificial fertilizers people were stuck with the natural. Yes, I am talking about manure. With the need for manure being high there was also a need to transport it. Thus the transportation of manure became a growing business. Eventually manure was even crossing large bodies of water, and this is where our story begins.

When the manure was transported onto the ship, it was logically shoveled onto the bottom floor of the boat to help contain the smell. Doing this became a problem. When you put a lot of manure into a confined space, that space becomes filled with flammable gasses. Eventually what would happen was some sailor would walk below deck with an open lantern and blow the ship to kingdom come. To prevent the unwanted explosions, the sailors would first dry the manure onshore. After the manure was dry it would be loaded below deck. This did not solve the problem. Boats of this age would inherently leak. This meant that the manure got wet, produced the gas, and eventually turned the ship into a floating powder keg. Finally, someone got wise and decided to package the dried manure into paper bags. The bags helped some, but the water could still seep through the paper, which meant that the manure would still get wet. In the end the bags that contained the manure needed to be placed on shelves while they sat below deck to keep the water away. In order for the crew to know which bags needed to be stored on shelves, sailors would write SHIP HIGH IN TRANSPORT on the bags of manure. Eventually the phrase was shortened to S.H.I.T.. Thus the word S.H.I.T. is a nautical term. Our story does not end here.

While at sea, if a ship's crew was not careful when handling their bags of S.H.I.T., the bag would rip and manure would fall from the shelves onto the floor. Once on the floor the manure would get wet, produce gas, and eventually blow the ship sky high. If there was a nearby ship that was able to witness the explosion, the captain would often yell out the cause of the explosion to his crew so they would not make the same mistake. What he would yell was "Holey S.H.I.T.". Notice the spelling of *holey*. Sailors, when returning home, would often use the same phrase when something bad would happen, but the public interpreted the phrase as holy shit, which really doesn't make sense to me. How can shit be holy?

Anyways, the next time something bad happens and someone gets angry at you for using Holey S.H.I.T., just tell them you're not swearing, you are just using an old nautical term, and if they tell you that you talk like a sailor you can tell them they are absolutely right! Let me end this story with the following: Holey S.H.I.T., I Had Cancer.

Brain Surgery

It's all about perspective. Each scar I now have I consider a badge of honor, and

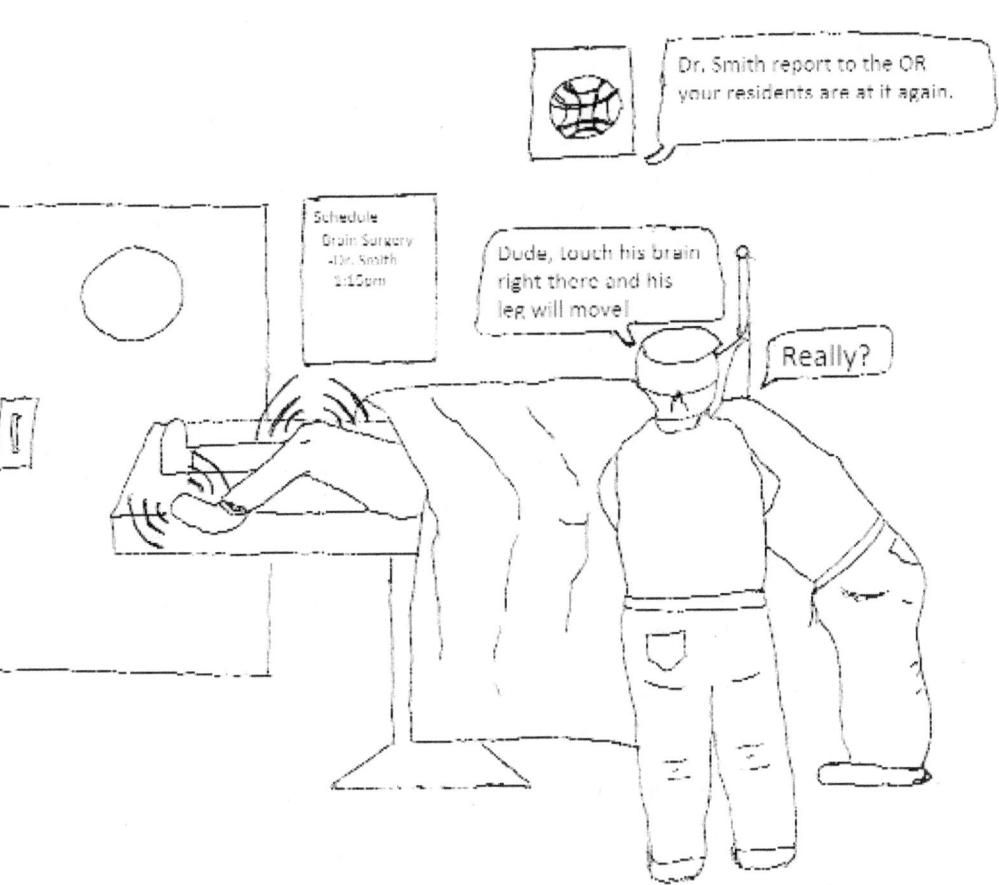

considering the total number of scars, I am a well-decorated, finely tuned soldier. My scars do not serve as reminders of my poor luck; instead, they demonstrate my perseverance and my endurance. They show that I can persevere through hard times. They show that I'm not a quitter. Again, when taking in the number of scars, I should be unstoppable. My medi-port serves the same purpose. Yes, I got to keep it and I still have it today. My medi-port is not a reminder of all the chemotherapy sessions. My medi-port is a reminder of what I can survive and accomplish. Again it's all about perspective. Its holey S.H.I.T. not holy shit.

On the other hand you can also use your scars to play with people. This can be a very enjoyable experience and I highly recommend it. If you are out swimming and some inquisitive person has to know how you got that scar on your chest, you tell them about the time you were in a knife fight. You let them know that you survived a stabbing to the chest while saving a little old lady from being robbed. Furthermore, if someone has to know how you got that horseshoe shaped scar on the top of your head, you tell them that you were once a jockey.

You tell them that on your last race, before you were forced to retire, you fell and got kicked in the head by your own horse. Sometimes the looks on people's faces can be priceless.

There was one event, while bald, where I did actually get to use my head, pun intended. This adventure involved me having to go to the dentist. You should know that I had come to form a strong relationship with the staff at the dentist office at this time in my life. As any kid who has braces knows, you spend a lot of time at the dentist office for things like broken rubber bands, wires needing trimmed, and so forth. After a while their entire office could have been supported simply from the revenue made for my orthodontic work. Well, that is what my dad liked to say. What made this visit to the dentist different was the fact I had not been there in a while and would have to remove my hat in order to be seen. At the time I never really liked taking off my hat in public. It made me uncomfortable. I had also noticed it could make other people uncomfortable as well. Some people had a hard time knowing what to do or what to say. What I ended up doing was taking some old face paint and having my mom paint a smiley face on the top of my head, but this was a special smiley face. Below the face's right eye was a horseshoe shaped scar where smiley got kicked by a horse! So I went to sit in the dentist chair with my hat on. I was asked if it would be okay to remove my hat. I said yes. I had to sit in a chair alone for the next ten minutes due to the fact that the hygienist had peed her pants. There still may be a Polaroid photo in the back of Dr. Hutchison's office that resembles an alien face smiling at you—an alien that was apparently kicked by a horse.

Now I would like to share one final thought about my head and being bald. The issue has now unexpectedly come full circle. What do I mean by this? Well, my hair grew back as expected when the entire cancer treatment process was over, but now, seventeen years later, it is starting to fall out all over again. Don't worry, this time it is due to male pattern baldness and I have my father's genes to thank for that. Within a few more years, hopefully not months, my scars will be visible again. Now I am starting to think what to do about this? My thinking now is that I would rather have my scars than the classic horseshoe shaped hair pattern. I'm actually thinking of shaving my head and going bald for the second time in my life.

Chemotherapy

If I'd never had cancer I would never have met Dr. Michael Wollman, and now is a good time to reintroduce him. Dr. Wollman comes into the picture after having brain surgery. He was my hematology oncologist, which basically meant that he was a specialist in the areas of blood and cancer. The two fit together in the sense that, when treating cancer, he prescribed drugs that were delivered via the blood stream and that most of the side effects of these drugs affect the blood. He also became my primary doctor throughout the entire cancer treatment process

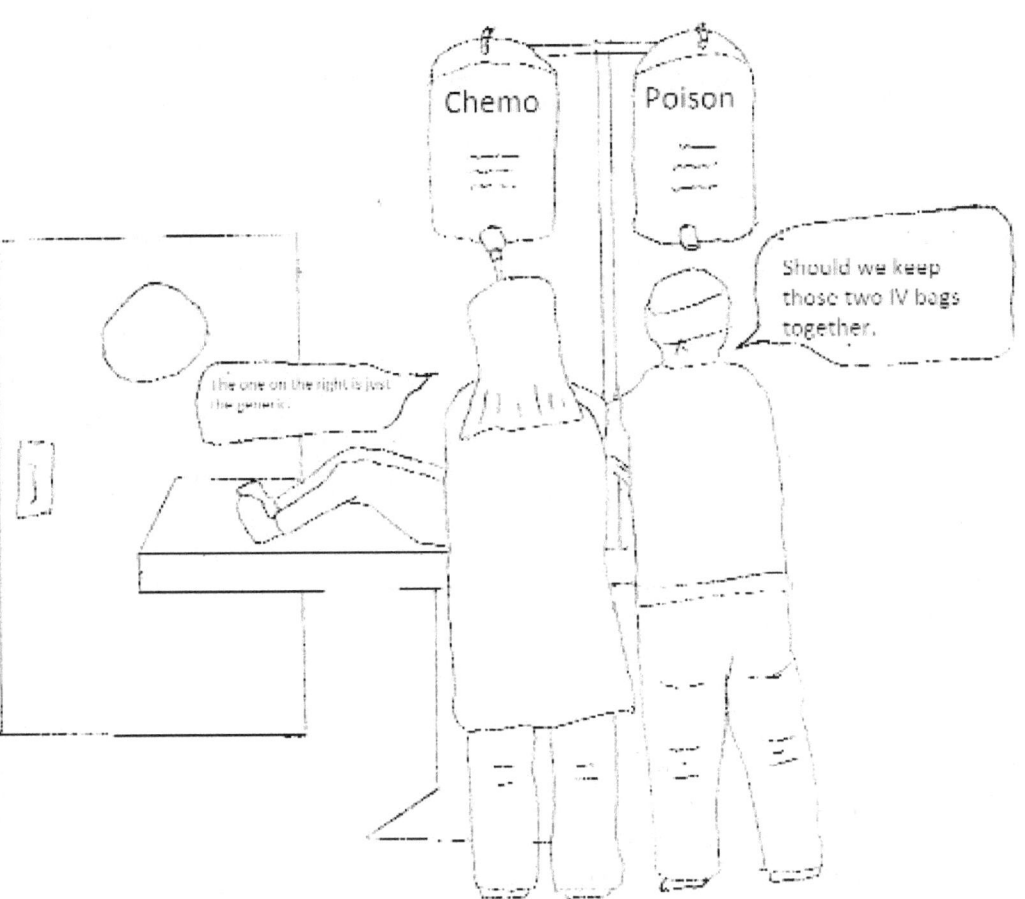

and was the doctor I would follow up with for the next ten years after treatment was over. It would be fair to say that we got to know one another. In life it is always good to find a few people that inspire you and that you can emulate. For me this was Dr. Wollman. What made Dr. Wollman great was that he was a good listener. In my case he quickly noticed my dry sense of humor and not only accepted it but tried to give it back. I would tease him and he would tease me in the same manner. Besides being kind, this man also recognized that I had an interest in science and a growing interest in medicine. This is where Dr. Wollman went above and beyond his role as a doctor and became a mentor. Whenever possible this man would keep me involved in the medicine of my own case. I remember when I was in the outpatient cancer center he always let me look at my own blood slides along with him. He would actually try to teach me when I was there. With a microscope we would evaluate my blood, looking at white cells, red cells, and platelets, but believe it or not, this is just the start of what Dr. Wollman did for me.

To graduate high school I had to do a senior graduation project and the topic I had chosen was pediatric cancer. This was something I knew well from the patient's prospective. To understand the doctor's point of view on the subject, Dr. Wollman was kind enough to let me shadow him for an entire week and again he took time to teach. He even let me participate in the oncology rounds with him and the residents at the hospital. I then got to follow up with his patients in the outpatient clinic. He embraced and nurtured my interest in medicine to the point that it became the driving force for applying to medical school. I did get into medical school and guess who wrote one of my letters of recommendation? Cancer is a disease that I never want to go through again, but my past with cancer is something I do not want to replace. Without this experience I would've never met Dr. Wollman and today I may not be enjoying my career as much as I do. As I write this I am a resident physician in the same hospital system as Dr. Wollman, and from time to time I am even able to stop by and say hi. Thank you, Dr. Wollman. Words are not enough to describe what you have done for me.

As I am writing about Dr. Wollman, another idea is forming in the forefront of my conscience. This idea concerns the art in medicine, and because it is stuck in my head I will talk about it now to get it unstuck. Diagnosing and prescribing treatment for a patient in and of itself is pretty black and white and requires little creativity. As a doctor you spend years learning how to properly evaluate symptoms in a standardized approach and then learn how those symptoms are related and come about. Once that is accomplished you simply attach the correct diagnosis (sometimes this is easier said than done). Once a diagnosis is made there is usually a standardized treatment protocol to be followed. Now this process does require an immense amount of knowledge but like I said it's pretty black and white. So, where is the color? Where is the creativity? Where is the art in medicine?

I would argue that most of the art in medicine lies in the interaction with the patient. A physician can respond to a patient in a number of ways and no particular way is always right. What is important is that the physician in some manner communicate to the patient that he or she has their best interest at heart, thus forming an element of trust in the relationship. Trust between patient and physician is key. Trust increases compliance with treatment and trust between physician and patient also prevents any under- or over-treatment as well. Under-treatment is avoided because the doctor is confident that the patient will follow protocols and not place themselves in harm's way. As a patient I always got my counts checked on time and if something came up I was always at the hospital for my IV urine. I did this because I trusted Dr. Wollman. To explain over-treatment, imagine a patient and doctor who come to an understanding or agreement of what is needed to be done. Now imagine that each party involved trusts that the other member will keep their word. If this occurs, the doctor no longer has to concern themselves with the big *what if.* This being, what if the patient does not show up next time and only needs to be prescribed the treatment or test most relevant at the time, thus preventing tests which later may be deemed unnecessary.

Unnecessary tests only expose patients to unnecessary side effects.

Now, establishing trust is easier said than done. To do this a physician must come to understand the values of an individual and learn how the patient interprets those values and chooses to express them. Thus at some level a doctor must establish empathy. This is not a bad thing. Physicians need to have some degree of empathy to understand their patients. Part of the art in medicine is to sense to what degree I must establish a connection with this patient to provide the best outcome for the patient and to a degree the physician as well. Every patient is different, and some interactions require more while others require less.

Having cancer had some positive experiences because certain doctors, who already knew what I needed, were able to read me and find a way to implement what was necessary. They recognized that I often used humor to handle difficult situations and understood this was how I coped. Knowing this they could easily speak to me and say what they needed to say. They also recognized a way to keep me moving in the right direction with my treatment plan. They found that I had an interest in science and, knowing that, involved me in the medicine of my own case. Ladies and gentleman, I propose this as the art of medicine. It is the creativity that one applies in order to establish a connection with the patient for their betterment.

Radiation

Once again, how we choose to remember an event can influence how we feel about it. For this reason I tell these next two stories. If you recall, for a period of time I had to drive an hour to the hospital every day, Monday through Friday, in order to receive radiation therapy. Neighbors would actually help out with the driving from time to time. One time in particular Mrs. Ramsey, the mother of one of my best friends Justin, drove Justin, another friend, and I down to the hospital, and on the way home she was going to take us out to lunch. Being young teenage boys the three of us joked about going to Hooters. Guess where Mrs. Ramsey took us when she overheard our conversation? This would be our first trip to this fine establishment for the three of us, and we would not be disappointed. Our waitress lived up to the restaurant's reputation. Now for the memorable part. It was my friend Ted who wanted to order wings but wanted them plain. To do so, according to the menu, he needed to say to the waitress, "I would like my wings naked." No matter how hard Justin and I would try, Ted could not do it. When I think about the period of time I spent being treated for cancer, I think about these memories and how Ted could not tell a half-naked woman that he would like his wings naked.

There was also another time when I recall the amazing Mrs. Ramsey driving me down to the hospital, only this time she drove the entire gang down with me. Those involve included Ted, Justin, my brother, Zach, Ted's two younger brothers, Jon and Chris, and Justin's younger brother, Ian. Now imagine trying to keep seven young boys in line while sitting in a hospital waiting room. Young

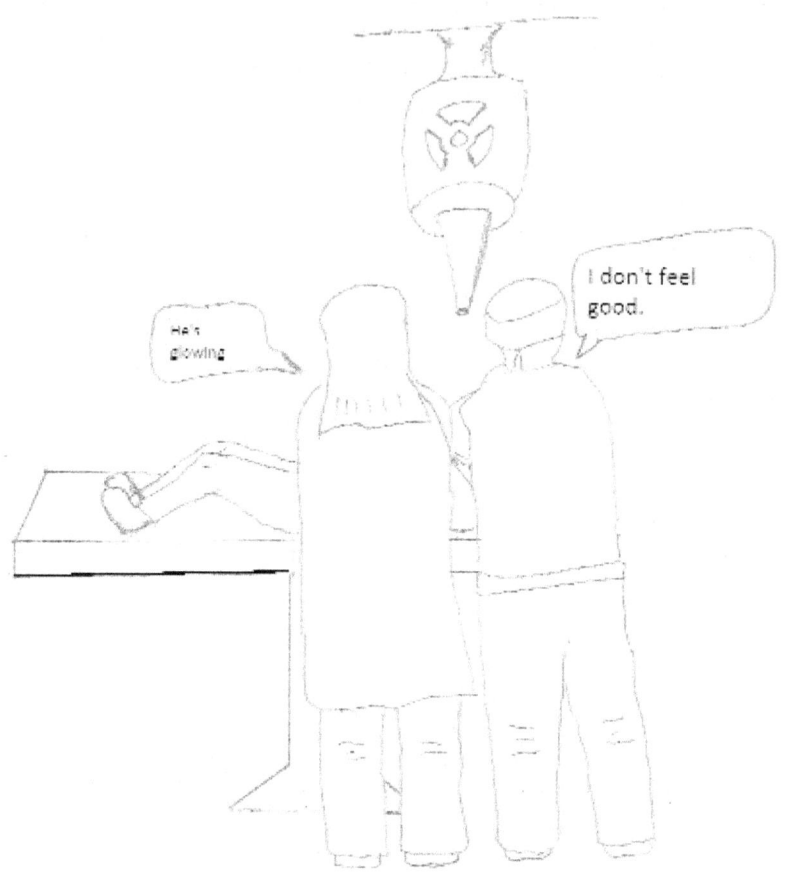

men congregating is not an unusual thing, but a hospital does not serve as the best location for such an event. As some of you may know when young men congregate a ritual event will begin to take place. It usually starts with one individual performing a small act of stupidity. Every other individual in the group than will try to outperform the previous act. Eventually it came to a climax and did so because one of us did something so stupid that Mrs. Ramsey put an end to it. I specifically remember on the way out the hospital door, Ian, the second youngest in the group, finding a foam cheese head in the garbage can, placing it on his head, and walking out the door. I say cheese head, but it was more like a disgusting piece of green foam. Where the foam came from I don't know, and we probably don't want to know. Ian didn't always think appropriately in his younger years. This is the only explanation I have for him doing this. We all tried to explain to him why you should not place a dirty piece of foam from the hospital garbage on your head. Ian survived but received a verbal lashing from our chaperone, Mrs. Ramsey, who was in fact his mother. Thank you, Mrs. Ramsey; you may be the only one who could do what you did.

The Hospital Staff

When you spend an entire year in and out of the hospital, you come to know the hospital staff, and if you let them the staff will come to know you. You will find that there are some people besides the doctors who truly take an interest in what happens to you. First and foremost are the nurses. They are the silent soldiers of the hospital and do most of the work when it comes to taking care of a patient. Even now, as a doctor, I will admit to this, but don't tell anybody, okay? As the primary caregivers in the hospital, due to the fact they do most of the work, nurses also have to deal with most of the crap in the hospital as well and this comes from everybody, patients, families, and, of course, the stubborn doctors. This crap can also be both figurative and literal by the way. In my professional opinion, thank God for nurses.

The first nurse I had when starting chemotherapy in the hospital was Julie. The simple fact that I can remember her seventeen years later must be a testament to her abilities. She was also the first person to have to access my medi-port; perhaps that factors in some. Two other nurses that I distinctly remember from the hospital are Rosie and Jason. Their names and faces are still ingrained in my head today simply due to the fact that they took good care of me despite me not always being the ideal patient. When I was in the outpatient clinic I always had the same nurse and she was the nurse. Her name was Donna. Whenever I was at the clinic, she was there as my nurse. Even when she moved on to a different position in the hospital as a research nurse, she came back to the clinic when I was there. Besides being a good caregiver, she became a good friend not just to me but to my parents as well. Having a good relationship with your nurse makes all the difference. This relationship may provide you with preliminary results on recent testing or may also give you first dibs on extra Jell-O sitting in the refrigerator. The special favors worked both ways. My parents and I were always willing to walk across the street (crossing the street now I always look both ways a few extra times to avoid any careless motorcyclists) to pick lunch up for Donna. Donna, if you ever read this, Thank you!

Another person I got to know well was one of the MRI technicians. The reasoning for this is simple. I had a brain tumor and everybody needed to look in my head, thus I spent a considerable amount of time in imaging. I must have had twenty or some scans in total. This woman was probably one of the most caring human beings that I ever met, and her name was Patty. We met her early on during my treatment when I was still bald and scarred. Initially, probably just by coincidence, she was the tech on when I first needed scanned, but as time passed, even when she was not the technician running my scan, she would always stop in to say hi to my parents and I when we were around. She always had a smile and gave everybody a hug. Becoming good friends with Patty had a few nice benefits as well. During one particular day my parents and I were waiting hours to get my

MRI scan. Things got backed up due to an emergency. We were still waiting five hours after my scan was supposed to start. Patty was working that day, unbeknownst to me, and was not even scheduled to run my scan. This woman eventually took time out of her own schedule to run my scan to get me on my way. Thanks, Patty—you're the best. FYI, I think Patty was also running my scan the day I vomited all over the MRI machine!

Post Treatment: Certified Hero

It turns out my cancer affected a lot of people. I began to learn this fact toward the end of my treatment. One random day, while home from the hospital, I received a large yellow envelope in the mail. In the envelope was a plaque which stated that a middle school class of North Allegheny School District in Pittsburgh, PA, had elected me their hero. I had no prior knowledge that I would be receiving this award, so it came as a surprise. In this envelope was also an essay written by my cousin, who nominated me. Apparently each student in the class wrote an essay nominating someone as a hero. The class then voted on who they thought should win the award. I am grateful to my cousin for writing such wonderful words about me. What soon became apparent to me was that my struggles turned out to be other peoples' struggles. Overcoming your hardship can inspire others, remember this. My cousin, Lauren, who wrote that wonderful essay, eventually went on to get her master's as a physician assistant and now works with an orthopedic surgeon.

I would also like to think that my experience with cancer influenced two other people close to me. As you now know, I am a resident physician. What you do not know is that my younger brother is as well. What caused him to choose this career path? Well, when the time came for him to write his application essays to medical school, guess what he wrote about? He wrote about the experiences he had when his brother had cancer. Further evidence I have to support my claim that I may have influenced my brother would be the fact that he chose the same field in medicine as I did. I also like to think I had some influence on my sister as well. Although I have no direct evidence linking my experiences with her current work in getting her master's as a physician assistant, I like to think it factors in somewhere. Why am I telling you all this? It is not only me using my past to shape my future. My experience became significant enough for other people to use it to shape their future as well. When you are fighting to keep your life ,you will find that you fight for more than just yourself.

My experiences also inspired my father. No, he did not become a doctor, but he used his talents and his own abilities to make a difference. He also did it at the most important level. He gave to the patients. About once a year the outpatient cancer center at Children's would send many of its patients to a camp along with their brothers and sisters so they could spend time together outside of the hospital. In order to accomplish this money needed to be raised. For a time my father, having the necessary business connections, stepped up to the plate and was able to set up a yearly golf outing large enough to produce the necessary funds. The outings were held in my hometown of Latrobe, Pennsylvania. You may be asking why we did not use a more prestigious course in Pittsburgh, but if you know anything about golf then I am sure you have heard of Arnold Palmer. Mr. Palmer, who is a cancer survivor, is a native of Latrobe and owns the local country club, and if you were at one of these outings you may have met him. So, in conclusion, each year the hospital sent one of the heme/onc doctors to give a speech telling those involved how they were helping the kids, but on the first year there was no doctor speaking. It was just me. I remember that speech well for one particular reason. It was the first time I ever saw my grandfather cry.

Post Treatment: Bill Cosby

Having cancer has gotten me a lunch at Hooters, a few good laughs, the ability to inspire, and a speaking position at a charity golf outing. Cancer has also allowed me to meet someone who was influential to me during this time. First let me set the scene. For about a two week period, while receiving radiation, I stayed at my grandparents' house. My grandparents lived much closer to the hospital and it gave my parents a break from driving. While living with my grandparents, I found this archaic machine known as a record player. Now I know what a record player is, but this one actually worked. In their collection of records were a few old Bill Cosby albums. I would actually sit and listen to those albums for hours on end. The bit I like the most was when Bill talked about the time he got his tonsils taken out and the subsequent hospital stay. It was a perfect description of how a child can view things in the hospital. He begins his story with the reasoning for needing a tonsillectomy. He was informed that his tonsils were the guards in his throat and that they were equipped with guns and bazookas to ward off any intruders via the throat. In Bill's case the doctor informed him that his tonsils had not only lost the battle but had defected to the other side and thus had to come out. Being a kid, surgery scared Bill, so then came the infamous lie he was told by all the grownups, and being a child he accepted it as truth. You're going to be able to eat all the ice cream you want. Fascinated with this idea he was relieved of any anxiety and came up with the following conclusion as he sang about the upcoming feast. His first bowl of ice-cream he wasn't even going to eat. He was going to smear it all over his body and, in his words, be the most beautiful chocolate sundae you have ever seen. The next part that I distinctly remember is when he called out to the orderly who did not give him a meal tray on the day of surgery saying, "Hey you….almost the doctor" (everyone in the hospital wears a white coat). The orderly informs Bill he couldn't eat because he was going to have surgery and might throw up if he does. Bill's response, typical for a young boy, was, I ate a frog once and I didn't throw up. Finally there is the climax when he greets his friend Johnson who had just come back from a tonsillectomy before he himself would have his surgery. He is now excited because after surgery it's time for ice cream. He runs over to his friend, looks at him and says, "Hey, Johnson...wake up.... (There is an ominous pause.) Seeing the blood in his mouth he says to the nurse, "Nurse, please tell me that's ketchup...that's ketchup, right?" Finally he comes to a conclusion, yelling, "Oh my God...they killed Johnson," and he breaks a bottle trying to use it to defend himself. Then he turns to the nurse when all else had failed and asks, "Would it mean anything if I told you I had breakfast?"

Upon awakening several hours later, Bill's parents try to get him to open his eyes. Bill couldn't do it. Every time he did the room acted silly. Nonetheless as he drifted back to sleep he mumbled the word i-c-e-c-r-e-a-m. The skit was good because it made me think about my own time in the hospital from a prospective that could make me laugh and it still does.

About a year after treatment, for Christmas my brother, sisters, and I got tickets to go see Bill Cosby, and guess who got to take us? If you guessed my grandparents you would be right. It was a good show, but the after show made my day. On the way out the door I had a revelation. In the lobby of the theater I found an event worker and told this person that I was a cancer patient and that I never got to make a wish, and if it was possible, could I at least say hi to Bill Cosby? The event worker was a little perplexed but said she would see what she could do. Within a few minutes my siblings and I were being escorted through the hallways of the theater. When I reached the room that he was in his first words were, "Is this him?" He was expecting me! I got to speak with him for about ten minutes. He was very nice. I got to talk to him about his tonsil's story and how it related to my time in the hospital. The answer I gave to one of his last questions was telling him that I was in remission from my cancer. His reply to my answer was, "No, son, you're in permission." Till this day I am not exactly sure what he meant. Perhaps he meant that I was given permission to live, which will bring me to another topic shortly.

The Evidence

This section is for all the skeptics who may think I am full of crap and would like some evidence. Now I could say to the skeptic, "Just take me at my word," but where is the fun in that. Luckily for all you skeptics, I have found some visual evidence to substantiate some of my claims. My hope is that this makes my story more real and helps to give you a better visual image of certain events. It took some ransacking of my old room at my parent's house and turning the closet in that room upside down, but I found four exhibits in total. I know it's only four, but remember this was sixteen years ago and the four that I did find are pretty good. First, I will give you some proof validating the motorcycle accident from when I was five. Then I will show you pictures I have taken of my medi-port and radiation mask. Finally I have a copy of the photo from the dentist office! Enjoy.

Exhibit A

What you are looking at is a newspaper clipping concerning my accident. Yes, after all these years I was actually able to dig this up. Can you believe it? This article on the day I scanned it was about twenty-four years old. It was found in an envelope in my mom's closet. Why she kept it all these years I really do not know, but I am glad she did. This means I get to share it with you. Reading this article brings one thing to mind, and that one thing concerns the adolescent who hit me. What does he look like? Does he remember the accident? What kind of person is he? What is he doing today? I never met this person nor have I ever seen what he looks like. I am only left to speculate. Maybe today he is a motorcycle safety instructor. Who knows? I will say that I hold no grudge or ill will towards this person. Why should I? What happened then was so long ago. Any effects from the accident have long since past or are so minor I don't notice them. In fact, today it serves best as a good story to tell.

> August 6 — .... was driven by Chad Kolas, Murrysville. Pedestrian involved was Matthew Walton, Murrysville. The accident occurred on Mayer Drive near Ivy Lane. Injured were taken to Forbes Health Center and Children's Hospital by Medic 1 and Lifeflight.

Exhibit B

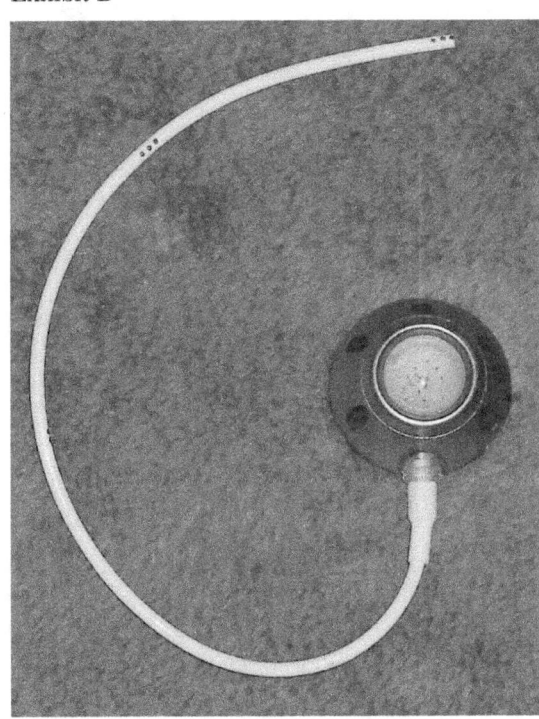

What you see here is my medi-port—not just any generic medi-port but the actual medi-port that was once inside me. On the day it was to be removed the surgeon asked if I wanted to keep it. Being me, a very inquisitive person, I immediately had to say yes. It now sits in my closet in a biohazard bag. The port was cleaned by the hospital, but they gave it to me in this bag and I have kept it in there ever since. If you recall I received my chemotherapy through this device. This saved the veins in my arms from countless pricks which inevitably would have destroyed my peripheral vasculature. The device sat underneath the skin on my chest. It was accessed by placing a needle through the skin and into the port. The white tube then connected the port to a vein which then carried the fluid and medicine to my heart to be pumped to the rest of my body. If you recall it was because of this device that I have a large scar on my chest. This scar I often refer to as my stabbing wound, which in a sense is true. After all, this wound was made with a scalpel.

Exhibit C

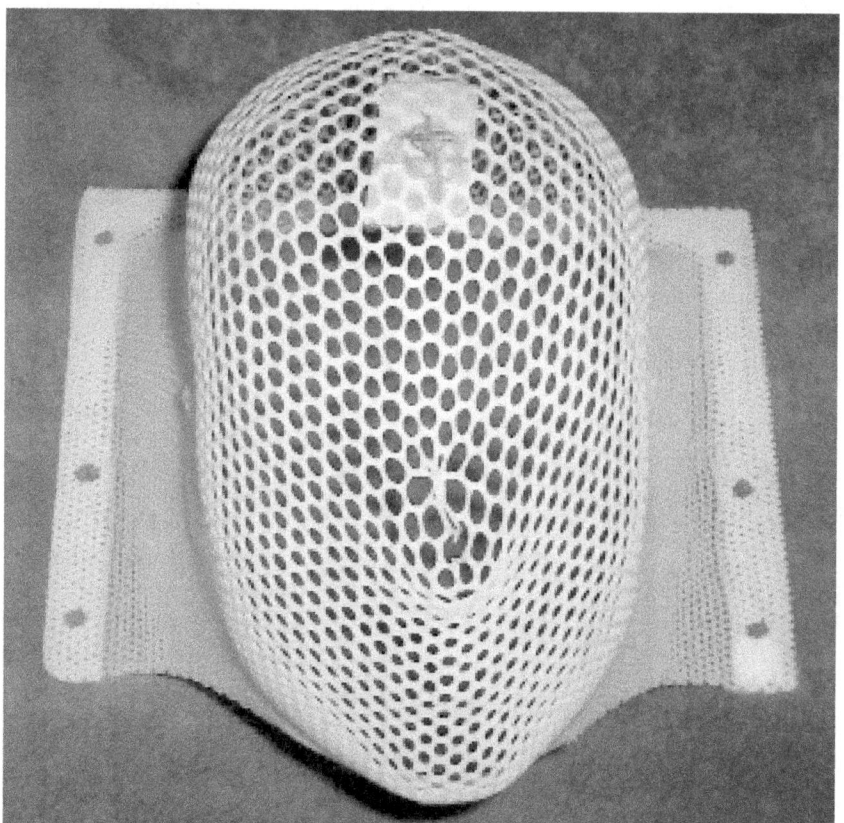

This is my radiation mask. Again when they asked if I wanted to keep it I had to say yes. Wouldn't you? It was custom molded to fit my face. That being said, it really doesn't fit any more. When I received radiation my head would sit on a tri-angular piece of foam. The mask would then be placed over my face and screwed into the table. Notice the holes; those are where the screws went. Several sides of the mask still have a piece of yellow tape with an "X" drawn on it. This is where they actually aimed the radiation. Speaking of radiation, it would be interesting to find out if this mask is radioactive. I doubt it, but if I could just get my hands on a Geiger counter.... On the day I took this picture the mask was about sixteen years old and I found out, after trying it on, that it is starting to dry out and break apart.

Exhibit D

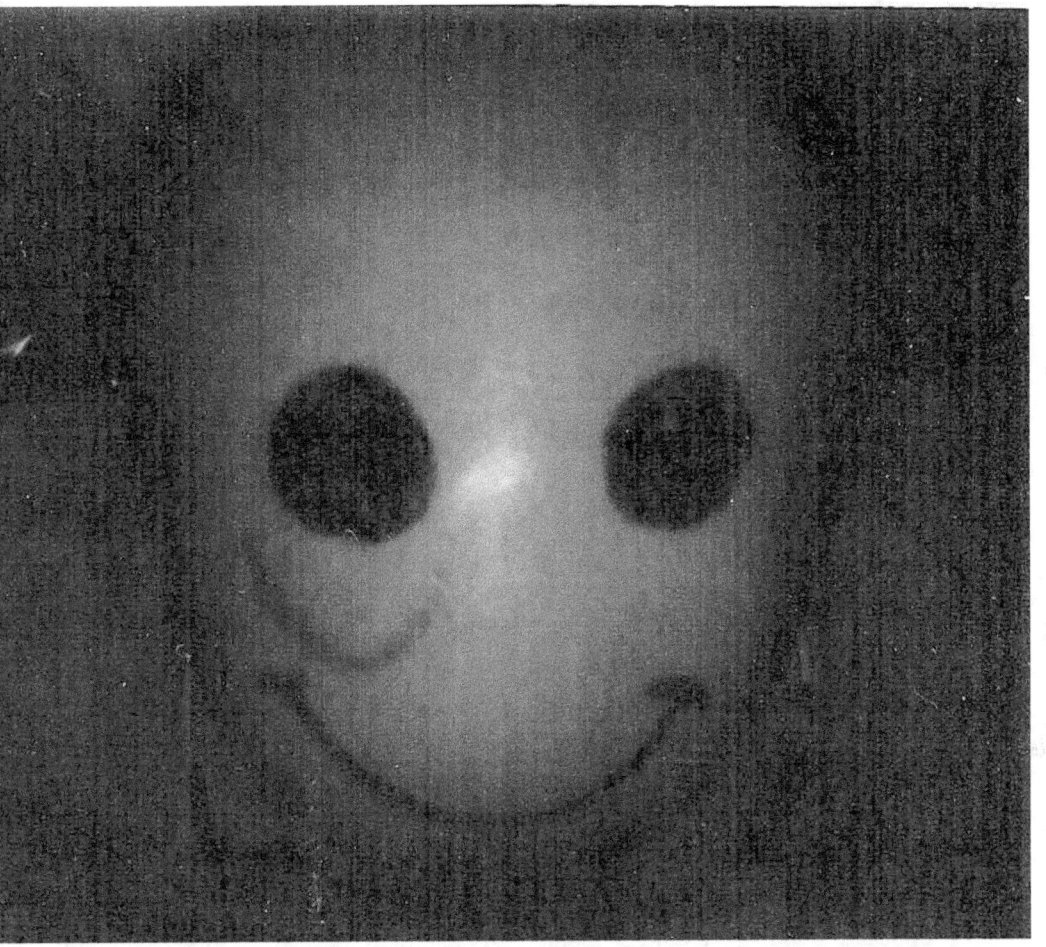

Okay, here it is, folks, the climax. I am saving the best for last. This is the alien that got kicked in the face by a horse. Yes, this is the picture taken at the dentist's office. This picture has not been altered in any way. For some reason only the top of my head stands out while the background got blacked out. They used a Polaroid camera that was adapted for taking pictures of dental work. It worked out perfectly. The head painting, if you recall was done by my mother. I told you she did a good job. (Thanks, Mom!) You will notice a scar underneath the right eye. This is the scar from the shunt/biopsy. This picture on the day I scanned it was about sixteen years old. Always try to find the happy face when you are in a dark place.

Part 3: Lessons
Hey, God, Are You There?
Science and God

Science has revolutionized the world and has had a significant impact on the world of medicine. Science has given us the ability to create vaccines and medicines to cure diseases that were once incurable. Science gives us the ability to create technology enabling us to replace organs with machines. Science gives us the ability to create the necessary imaging and the know-how to remove a tumor from the middle of someone's brain. As a doctor I now work in a field that demands I think scientifically. A doctor's reasoning is based on research and what we have learned about life through trial and error. For some there is only a God of the gaps. It seems logical to say that science is replacing God, that there is no need for a god when we can seemingly explain and accomplish all these things with science.

There is an error with the preceding hypothesis. Science describes mechanisms or processes. In turn this gives us the ability to make predictions of what will happen. Science describes the process but says little about the process itself. For example, where did the process come from? Charles Darwin postulated the theory of evolution, and we can use his theory to illustrate this point. Darwin, in fact, did come up with a theory that describes a process. That process would be evolution. So far, in all respects, Darwin's theory is doing well and works well. It has given biologists a system to work with and enables them to make predictions. It gives us a tool to shape our future. Darwin's theory begins to lose credibility when some go on to explain the origin of the process, something science can't really do. Nevertheless they state that there was no real origin and the process is random and unguided. By stepping outside the bounds of science with this idea, you are now implicating some profound possibilities. If life did, in fact, evolve from a random unguided process, then who and what you are is meaningless. There is also the implication that you know nothing about yourself. A random unguided process says that the universe is not rational which in essence means that science is not possible. If science is not possible, why have a theory in the first place?

The point is, science explains how things work. It describes the process or mechanism. The existence of God explains why the process is there and works the way it does. Science and God go hand-in-hand and are not contradicting. To understand the universe's natural processes is to better understand God. This argument has been around for at least two thousand years, and I will prove it to you. The first chapter in the Gospel of John is testament that the early Christians were well aware of this concept. In the very first few sentences you learn the origin of the process. "In the beginning was the Word (the Logos) . . . " (John 1:1).

"As a man who has devoted his whole life to the most clear headed science, to the study of matter, I can tell you as a result of my research about atoms this much: There is no matter as such. All matter originates and exists only by virtue of a force which brings the particle of an atom to vibration and holds this most minute solar system of the atom together. We must assume behind this force the existence of a conscious and intelligent mind. This mind is the matrix of all matter."

-Max Planck

God and I

Early in my diagnosis, the most frequent conversation I had with God was, *Why me?* More specifically, I was adamant on knowing why God would let this happen to me. I am referring to the whole cancer thing, in case you forgot. I was a decent person. At least I thought so. Things like this are not supposed to happen to good people, right? It appeared that God was just a mean kid who had a magnifying glass pointed at me on a sunny day, but as I grew older I grew out of this point of view and would now strongly argue against it. The big question though still remains. Why do things like cancer affect innocent people? The following is how I have come to answer this question. God has given us all a gift and that gift is life. Each of us are given a finite period of time to exist within the material universe. During this time we are subject to no one and we are capable of influencing our surroundings to whatever end we choose. Take a minute to think about that. Now if God, a sentient being, made the universe he would have had to make it in such a way so that everything would work in harmony. We all know the universe is a vast place. A place where trillions upon trillions of reactions take place every instant. Some of those reactions take place within our very own cells. Most of the time these reactions are beneficial for us or we would not exist. However, on rare occasions a reaction must occur within us that is not beneficial to us but is necessary to balance the greater equation of the universe and sometimes this will result in a disease that we had no part in obtaining. Put another way, if you are to live within this universe there are certain potential consequences that you must accept. Next question, if God does not work in the material world, how can he act? The answer is simple. He works in the immaterial.

Let's go back to that first night I was receiving chemotherapy in the hospital. It was the middle of the night and I was lying in bed. While staring at the ceiling I prayed to God asking him to spare my life. Did God do anything? While there was no visible or material event that night that I can point to proving a miracle I believe God did act. Oftentimes in our everyday life we neglect to see the Lord before us. When life is good we are blinded to the acts of the Almighty. It is only when we are down and in need of tremendous help that we can feel God's presence in front of us. Bill Cosby's Noah serves as a perfect example. Even when God speaks to Noah directly and tells him he is the Lord Noah's response is," Yeah, right."

When I asked for God's help, he did not respond in the material, making the tumor disappear; instead, he worked in the immaterial. One of the gifts that God bestows upon each and every one of us is the Holy Spirit and though it is one spirit it presents in many forms and those that possessed the skills necessary to cure my illness God placed before me. My neurosurgeon was at the top of his field. To emphasize this fact I remember having an appointment with him canceled due to the fact that he was lecturing in Poland. I also had Dr. Wollman, who I can best describe as a great doctor and a wonderful human being. There were also the nurses who day in and day out worked with diligence and compassion. This is what God did.

Did God do anything else on that fateful night? To answer my own question, I think he did. Over the past few years I have come to understand that when we truly need it and ask for the extra strength to get through an adversity God will provide. You just have to ask. I believe this is what happened on the night I asked for help. Another concept that I have come to understand is that whatever extra God provides in your time of need he does not take back.

"And the God of all grace, who called you to his eternal glory in Christ, after you have suffered a little while, will himself restore you and make you strong, firm and steadfast" (1 Peter 5:10).

This extra strength remained with me and led me to get my medical degree, or osteopathic degree, to be more precise. I was never the smartest or in the top 10% of my class. This is true for high school, college, and medical school, but I was always being pushed by some invisible force. I was always striving to better myself. There was a fire within me that kept burning even in the dark and difficult times and there were many of them. I lit that fire, but God saw to it that the fire never went out. He nurtured that flame. He always made sure there was enough fuel. At times when it felt like I should quit he may have also thrown some gasoline in for good measure. God is always willing to work with you. You just have to be willing to work with him.

Talking to God

The power of prayer is immense. When I was sick I literally had people from around the world praying for me. This was mainly due to my Uncle Bobby, aka Fr. Jude, a Catholic priest and Carmelite. I will tell you that just knowing the simple fact that there were people praying for me from around the world did wonders for my psyche. Can you imagine? There were complete strangers out there speaking to God on my behalf. How cool is that?

So, what is prayer? To me, prayer, in its most basic essence, is you opening up to God. Prayer does not have to be a ritualized saying. Just start talking to God. Tell him about your day. Tell him what you think. You can argue with God, just do so fairly. There is one story in the Bible that I would like to use to emphasize this point. It starts with Abram—yeah, that guy from the Old Testament. He pleaded with God not to destroy Sodom and Gomorrah so that innocent people could be saved namely his nephew Lot. After some discourse God listened to what Abram had to say and because of this the innocent were taken from the city before it was destroyed. What I take from this story is that God does not just hear us but listens to what we have to say. Now, a final point about arguing with the Almighty. A true argument is a means to an end. Here that end is an understanding of why things are the way they are. A true argument with the Lord can help us to come to an understanding with whatever adversity we encounter. Think about it.

If you have trouble starting a conversation with God, one prayer I know well is the prayer of St. Francis of Assisi. I like it because it asks God to do what he does best, to work through us. It does not ask God to make something appear or disappear. Instead it asks God to show us the gifts within us. It asks God to let us be the miracle.

Lord, make me an instrument of your peace.
Where there is hatred, let me sow love;
where there is injury, pardon;
where there is doubt, faith;
where there is despair, hope;
where there is darkness, light;
and where there is sadness, joy.
O Divine Master, grant that I may not so much seek
to be consoled as to console;
to be understood as to understand;
to be loved as to love.
For it is in giving that we receive;
it is in pardoning that we are pardoned;
and it is in dying that we are born to eternal life.

Death

A conversation between a medical student and a man dying of cancer:

Student: "Death. To die. To expire. To pass on. To perish. To peg out. To push up daisies. To push up posies. To become extinct. Curtains, deceased, demised, departed and defunct. Dead as a doornail. Dead as a herring. Dead as a mutton. Dead as nits. The last breath. Paying a debt to nature. The big sleep. God's way of saying, Slow down."

Patient: "To check out."

Student: "To shuffle off this mortal coil."

Patient: "To head for the happy hunting ground."

Student: "To blink for an exceptionally long period of time."

Patient: "To find oneself without breath."

Student: "To be the incredible decaying man."

Patient: "Worm buffet."

Student: "Kick the bucket."

Patient: "Buy the farm."

Student: "Take the cab."

Patient: "Cash in your chips."

Student: "And if we bury you ass up, I have got a place to park my bike."

-*Patch Adams*, the movie, 1998

We often think of death as the end, the point at which our prospective into the future comes to an end. What we neglect to realize is something that science has taught us about the mechanism. We all learned this in elementary physics, and I am sure the concept is ingrained somewhere in your mind. We know that for every action there is an opposite and equal reaction. What does this mean? It means nothing in this universe ends. It is only transformed. All of the energy/matter that existed at the beginning is here today in one form or another. Some of that energy is used to make you and one thousand years ago part of that same energy was used to make someone else. Part of what is you today will be part of someone else in the future. Our physical self is in essence immortal and it will never vanish. Perhaps God is trying to teach us something.

The soul and the body are similar in many respects. Both are eternal in their own right and both have existed since the beginning. However, as the body transforms the soul does not. The soul is the part of you that remains constant just as God does. Your soul starts in heaven with God and there you are given a gift, a gift of physical life. You are placed in the physical world and bound by its natural constraints but you are otherwise free to change things as you see fit. Perhaps this is God's way of bringing us closer to him by giving us a freedom that God may have only once had. Death is the point when the soul is separated from this godlike status. Perhaps this is why we have such a hard time with it.

With this framework in mind, I will try to answer the following question. Why would God let a child die from cancer or why would God take the gift of life away so early? I believe there's a point when God sees that his gift is no longer a gift and a person's suffering is outweighing any foreseeable benefit. At this point, I believe God would rather have that person returned to him in paradise. How can I best describe paradise or heaven? Heaven is our true home. It is where we are meant to be. Here we can receive the greatest comfort there is. The good book tells us that Jesus is waiting in heaven and has prepared a place for each and every one of us. If someone close to you has been taken too early, always keep this in mind. It can help you make the correct choices in life because the correct choices will lead you to an eternal life with your friend.

Miracles

As I said before God regularly works through the immaterial or through created nature, yet he is free to work without it, above it, or against it. Remember that point when a person's suffering outweighs any foreseeable benefit? At this point God will usually take us from the suffering, but on rare occasions God may just remove the suffering. When this happens the event is often referred to as a miracle. Miracles best serve as a constant reminder that God is still with us in the physical world. Miracles imply something very profound. During the brief instant when the miracle occurs there is a violation in the laws that govern the universe. What does this mean? In essence, the entire universe is placed on hold. Imagine, God will place the entire universe on hold for a single individual.

Miracles are rare events, and they have to be due to their severe magnitude or implications. If miracles were to occur on a regular basis there would be no universal laws. Without these laws there would be no science and again we would have the complications described earlier. Miracles are rare, but they do happen. One way to demonstrate this point is trying to follow the number of people canonized every year. For each and every person elected a saint, he or she must have at least two miracles attributed to them. The point here is that with God nothing is impossible and everything is possible. With this said I would not go through life expecting God to violate his own natural laws. Instead I would say to ask God to work through you with the gifts that he gave you. This may not prove to others that God exists but it will provide you with a closer relationship to God. A closer relationship with God can lead you to a place where miracles become the natural law.

Purpose

"Why do you do it? Why get up? Why keep fighting? Do you believe you're fighting for something? For more than your survival? Can you tell me what it is? Do you even know? Is it freedom? Or truth? Perhaps peace? Yes? No? Could it be for love? ... Why? Why do you persist?"

—Agent Smith, *Matrix Revolutions*

Why talk about purpose?

I am speaking about purpose because this is what cancer gave me. I find it amazing how something with such morbidity and mortality can do something so powerful, but first let me explain why purpose is so important. Just as God answers the why when it comes to the universe purpose answers the why when it comes to how you relate to the universe. Purpose though is more than just the principal of satisfying your immediate needs. It is more than just survival. Survival has the potential to confine us. Purpose has the ability to set us free. This is why purpose is so important. Purpose helps to aim our lives in one direction or another. Purpose gives us a path in life and gives us the strength to continue on that path. It puts reasoning into the choices we make. Living with purpose gives life meaning. This is why I am talking about purpose and why purpose is so important. It will help define you. It will help to characterize you.

Another important concept about purpose is the following. If you recall, the universal laws were bestowed upon us by a higher power. Purpose is different in this respect. It is something we must bestow upon ourselves. There is no assembly line in heaven where every soul is assigned a purpose. Angels do not come down from heaven and shove a purpose into our heads. Neither can we earn purpose. God will not reward us with a purpose for a good deed. We were born with free will. We get to choose what to do and what not to do. You can think of purpose as the meaning of life. I know this is a bold statement, but think about it from another angle. You must find purpose to give life meaning.

"Destiny is not a matter of chance; it is a matter of choice. It is not a thing to be waited for; it is a thing to be achieved.

—William Jennings Bryan

How to Obtain Purpose

Now that we have become educated on the importance of purpose, we can continue. Like I said before, purpose is something we must plant within ourselves. It is the proverbial mustard seed. Just as faith brings us closer to God, purpose will bring us closer to ourselves. The Bible used the mustard seed as a way to describe faith. It was the smallest known seed at the time and the people knew it had the potential to produce something very large and hard to control. The mustard plant was a malignant weed with dangerous take-over properties. The same is true with purpose. Purpose has the potential to enable us to do so much, but its origins begin with the simplest of ideas and once those ideas are ingrained action is inevitable.

Purpose is derived from imagination and imagination is derived from inspiration. In other words inspiration is the stimulation needed for creative thought. That stimulation starts early. As children our minds are open. We are blank slates or a canvas waiting to become a masterpiece. Inspiration will come from every direction. It starts simple with the senses. We see, hear, touch, and feel new things all the time. I guess you can put taste in there as well, but we don't experience every new event with our tongue out. These new sensations we often cannot describe, hence they stimulate the imagination. As we grow so does that which inspires us. As the mind takes precedent over the senses it is the concept of an idea that begins to inspire us.

When we are filled with inspiration we begin to imagine what we can do. As children our imagination takes us to the limit of possibility and perhaps beyond. Young boys imagine being superheroes and young girls imagine being princesses. As we mature, so does our imagination. There will come a point when you begin to see what you're imagining is possible. When this time comes and you choose to chase this dream, you now do so with purpose.

As I grew up many of the people around me who received respect were those involved in the care of others. I noticed that their acts would benefit others but they too would inherently benefit from the same act. When I began to imagine, my dreams were as a superhero of sorts, a cosmic white knight. I would travel to far-off lands or to a parallel universe to engage evil in battle, and even though my powers were cosmic in nature I often only needed a shield and sword. I specialized in the conquering of dark warlords, demons, and emperors. As I grew up so did my dreams, but my dreams did not change—they only matured. The White Knight slowly morphed into something else, and this is when purpose was sparked into existence. The armor of the White Knight began to morph into the fabric of the white coat. That first night of chemotherapy was the night when I started to develop a purpose. I saw the people around me, those who were taking care of me, those who were doing it in such a specific way. I was inspired and I was imagining and I began to realize. As I said before, a fire was sparked into existence that night.

Benefits of Purpose

This fire became a beacon that guided me through life. This beacon kept me on the right path even when the path proved to be steeper and a whole heck of a lot longer than anticipated. The beacon of purpose reminds us why we are doing what we are doing. Its light makes are destination visible in the distance. It keeps us focused on the goal and not on the hardships of obtaining that goal, and when we reach that destination it gives us the confidence of knowing this is where we belong. There is confidence because of everything you had to endure to get there. In other words, purpose gives your accomplishments meaning because there is reasoning behind it.

When what you do has meaning, it no longer is work. It becomes part of what and who you are. This is what it means to love what you do. I will paraphrase my father here; when you do what you love you never work a day in your life. I am not a doctor because I enjoy working with stool, urine, blood, vomit, pus, sweat, boogers, earwax, spit, fungus, bacteria, viruses, prions, tears, screaming, foul smells, endless forms, and insurances. I am a doctor because it gives my life meaning and there is meaning because there's purpose.

The Lack of Purpose

There is a plague of sorts spreading throughout society. Unlike plagues of the past, this one stems more from indifference then from disease. Today one person has the ability to do what was once only possible with large groups of people. Where many were once needed to achieve a goal now we only need a few. In this regard modern society has blessed us. Now there should be more individuals each with their own purpose trying to have an impact on society. Society now has the potential to evolve exponentially, but as I said before there is a growing problem and we are all guilty of this to some degree. We are relying on the few because we can. It is now easier than ever to go through life without purpose simply using others to keep you at the status quo. Going through life without purpose is much like having a disease and not caring whether you get better, and if we don't want to get better we never will.

Going through life without purpose is a disease state much like cancer. You will go through life not having the control you need. This leads to the perception that life is controlled by external forces resulting in the conclusion that your life is not your own. Also, without purpose there is no focus. Without focus you are more susceptible to outside influences and the reasoning for doing things is also perceived as external. When something is accomplished based on external reasoning, there is often no real reward. If there is a reward, it is often immediate and short-lived. Find purpose.

"There is no escaping reason, no denying purpose. Because as we know, without purpose, we would not exist. It is purpose that created us. Purpose that connects us. Purpose that pulls us. That guides us. That drives us. It is purpose that defines us. Purpose that binds us."

—Agent Smith, Matrix Reloaded

Humility

"Humility is the foundation of all the other virtues hence, in the soul in which this virtue does not exist there cannot be any other virtue except in mere appearance."

--Saint Augustine

What is humility?

If you are reading the above quote and find it familiar, you are not mistaken and quite observant, I might add. I wish to return to the concept of humility. Humility is an old concept. Many of the proverbial teachings that have survived since antiquity are related to the topic of humility. You can go as far back as Confucius. Even he has something to say on the topic. You will also find that almost every culture has something to say about humility as well. Humility is a fundamental part of almost all the world's religions. You will find it in Buddhism, Hinduism, Islam, Sikhism, Judaism, and Christianity. Now in modern times, Webster and friends define humility as the act of being humble. If memory serves me right, according to the laws of grade school, at least at Mountain View Elementary, you cannot use the word you are defining in a definition. I define humility has acting on the concept that you are no better or no more important than anyone else. There is an important idea here. Did you catch it? Humility is more than just a concept or noun. It's a verb. There is no being humble. Instead you must act to be humble. Talking the talk does not cut it. You have to walk the walk and you can tell by the way you use your walk if you are a humble man no time to talk.

Why talk about humility? I am assuming that it would be easy to understand how cancer can relate to humility. Cancer is probably one of the most humbling experiences that you can live through. At least it was for me. When I was diagnosed with cancer I quickly came to the realization that my survival was dependent upon others. My ego had to give way, which meant there could be no pride. Pride is a bad thing. Please do not wait until you get cancer to learn this fact. Pride is the opposite of humility and is one of the proverbial seven deadly sins. Humility is one of the seven heavenly virtues, and it is specifically placed opposite of pride. This virtue, if upheld, leads us away from pride. So why am I talking about pride? I am talking about pride because of purpose.

If you have discovered your gifts and are using them to accomplish goals with a set purpose you are well on your way, but moving through life with just purpose can potentially cause us to move through life without conscience. Purpose is powerful and we must move through life with it but we must do so with humility and in that way we become the best all-around person we can. This is why I believe humility is so important. Simply stated, humility keeps us in balance. It keeps us in check. Some people take the idea of humility even further. For example there is St. Augustine who believes so much in the concept of humility that he proposes that it serves as the foundation for all other virtues.

A Further Review of Humus

Before I go any further, I know what you're thinking. You may be thinking, *What in the hell is humus?* but you may also be thinking that humility is equivalent to servitude. Please don't think of humility as servitude. Humility does not mean making others more important than you. It means making yourself no better than anyone else. Humility is following the golden rule. It is treating others the same way you would want to be treated. It is the second greatest commandment, to love your neighbor as yourself. Okay, back to the humus.

What is humus and why am I talking about it? I'm talking about humus because humility is derived from this word. At least I think it is. Humus is soil that has come to a point of stability and will not break down any further. Meaning it will not change. Humus significantly improves the soil structure and contributes to moisture and nutrient retention. Now that we have learned what humus is let us ask how humility is derived from humus. Humility is something that significantly improves the soul. Humility provides stability for the soul. It allows for the absorption of positive attributes. Humility is the humus which rests and all good humans.

The End

This may be abrupt but my story ends here. Why you ask? Well, I believe I have accomplished what I have set out to do. I have recalled all the events concerning a specific time in my life that I wished to analyze. I have summarized how I believe those events have affected me and finally have processed what I have learned. Now I'm sorry but this is where I will leave you but please don't cry. I hope you enjoyed or got something from my ramblings. I think I did. Now, being the intelligent person you are you may be asking yourself, if I'm done writing, why there are more pages. The proceeding pages are written by my father. When I started writing I thought it would be kind of cool to get someone else's point of view on everything that happened to me. My dad always talked about writing a book, so I asked him to contribute to this one and he agreed. I basically told him that I was writing about my experience with cancer and what I learned from it and gave him free rein. So without further ado, may I present my father.

Oh, sorry, one more thing. I can assure you that these are my father's words—I may have done some minor rearranging of paragraphs and sentences to make things flow a little better, but everything written here is my father talking. For the few places where I needed to say something I put it in brackets.

\

MY FATHER
Preface

It has been seventeen years since we found out my son Matthew had cancer. This past year he said he wanted to write a story about his experience and asked me to add a part from my perspective. I found this to be a bit difficult for a couple of reasons. First, I've never written anything, and second, I wasn't sure I wanted to reach back into that period of my life. Matt was pretty persistent and it seemed important to him, so I accepted the challenge.

At first I did not even know who my audience was or what presence I should write it in. After a while I thought maybe I should write this to other parents who are undergoing the same thing we did seventeen years ago. Maybe it might give them some of that hope Dr. Wollman taught me about. I also realized I wanted, and maybe this is the most important part, to thank all those who made this story into something positive for me and my family. If it does any of that then I have been victorious. Lots of the facts might be off, some off the important details I have forgotten entirely and don't appear here at all, and it doesn't matter. What does matter is the way people can come together in times of great upheaval and turmoil in their lives; to know that a son can teach you more about life than you could have ever found on your own; to know that overcoming great adversity is a part of living and should be celebrated every chance you get.

The Story

My memory when it comes to the details has faded a bit, and I think that is the way it is supposed to be. It was a Saturday morning when Matt was on the couch complaining about a headache he'd had for about three days. There was something different about the way he acted, which led us to decide to take him to the pediatrician. The pediatrician was located some fifteen miles away in Irwin, PA. My wife was in charge of all checkups, ear aches, and sore throats, so this one was mine. We called ahead and we headed off. Dr. Trainer was the doctor on call that weekend and there was nothing that was in my mind that this wasn't going to be any different than the seemingly 20,000 other visits we made.

It did not take long for Dr. Trainer to zero in on Matt's eyes. I thought that was curious as we had noticed that something was different but we did not connect any dots. We had taken a trip down the Youghiogheny River the weekend before and one of our close friends said something about his eyes. We just chalked it up to puberty or even bad habits he developed. The doctor asked Matt to look up, which he could not do. He asked him to follow the light which he could do in every other direction. I still didn't think anything was wrong. The doctor disappeared for a few minutes and came back in and repeated the same steps again. He had picked up a sense of urgency. Now I knew this wasn't typical, but still I never felt there was anything serious. He again disappeared and this time the look on his face had changed when he returned.

He looked at Matt and then addressed me. "Mr. Walton, I don't know what is causing Matt's eyes to not react or why he can't look up. I have scheduled you a CAT scan at Children's Hospital in Pittsburgh. They are expecting you, and I told them you would be there with in the hour. Do you have any questions?"

I felt the hair standing up on the back of my neck; I replied, "No," and headed out for Pittsburgh. I really don't remember the ride or if Matt and I discussed anything. It was a ride we were to repeat many times.

When we arrived at Children's we parked in the underground garage, and the first thing I noticed was a very pungent smell that I could never identify. I hated that smell. It's a smell that to this day could take me back to a lot of memories I'm not sure I want to have back. It was always a powerful reminder of all the good things and all the bad. Children's Hospital has since moved to a more modern and spacious building without the smell. I wonder if anybody else thought about that. I'm sure all the employees hated it. [*I remember this smell as well. It was even there when I was five and being treated for all my broken bones. It smelled like some of those degreasing agents you will find at an auto mechanic's shop.*]

I had been fortunate all my life in that I had not spent a lot of time in hospitals. Nonetheless I thought I could turn on my internal manly directional finder to get to Radiology. For some reason hospital walls had an effect and I couldn't find anything. I even broke down and started asking people how I get there. They seemed confident, but I could tell they thought I was a lost cause. Maybe the doctor should have told them I would be there in two hours. It turns out there was a confused architect that attached an old building to a newer one. The seventh floor on the old one was really the fourth floor on the new one. I know the numbers I'm giving are not right, but for sure I was not the only one who got lost in this hospital.

Radiology was not crowded. As soon as we arrived they took us to the CT scanner just as Dr. Trainer promised. They did the obligatory tests, we signed some papers and they put Matt in the machine. A CAT scanner gave you slices or pictures at different depths. I was standing where the images were coming up showing Matt's brain. It didn't take long and I could see the tumor behind his eyes. The technicians and nurses immediately changed their demeanor. They got on the phone and asked for the neurosurgeons to come to radiology stat. We didn't get the attending doctor; instead, we got the residents. They quickly huddled up and we became their next challenge in their career development. When they turned around to talk to us they forgot to remember we were human beings. They just told us Matt had a tumor and we would have to come back Monday.

That was it. Come back Monday.

I called my wife in almost disbelief. It was then I realized everything was about to change. The fog started to come over me. I prayed for God's help. The ride home was long. I stared at Matt a lot as he was relatively calm and he had a few questions I couldn't begin to answer. The thought I couldn't get out of my head was that I would never get through Sunday to get Matt back to the hospital on Monday.

When you get bad news you call your family, friends, and neighbors. Our lives were blessed with people that care and we leaned on them right away. Maybe it spreads out the anxiety, I don't know, but the leaning would get heavier and thank God all were there. Some never knew they helped me, and that's a reason for writing this story. Sometimes it is funny who you turn to for help.

One day I was on my way to work and I was struggling. I felt the need to reach out to someone who might understand what was going on. I pulled the car over to the side of the road and dialed a work friend of mine whose wife had just passed away from cancer. His name is Ted Gawel. Ted was always an upbeat person, but the death of his wife was tragic and I knew he was struggling too. When I called him I actually couldn't talk for a couple of seconds as I was choked up. I remember stammering and my mind was racing trying to come up with something to say. I told him that he was the only person I knew who had gone through the cancer experience and I was reaching out to him because I thought he might understand how I felt. I know I rambled on aimlessly bearing my soul. I don't think I let him say a word. Ted was a good listener and we would talk fairly often over the next several years. He was not a family member or a friend I saw often but somebody I could go to that cared and had been there before. He could always cheer me up.

Monday morning didn't come soon enough. Waiting was not one of my strong points, and in this story as I was about to learn it was all about waiting. I used the line hurry up and wait a thousand times over the next year. It was just how things worked in a hospital. You get used to it. Our appointment was with Dr. Albright, head of neurosurgery at Children's. He seemed a bit quirky. That was my first impression. I would learn as time went by that Dr. Albright was the smartest man to whom I ever had the privilege to talk. He had an unusual ecliptic way of talking. Pausing between each sentence, he seemed to want to say things in a way I would understand versus the way he converses with his peers. He measured every breath, with the exhale being the most important part. When I think about it with his job he dealt with life and death every day. I guess it was his way of communicating, slow and deliberate. He stared at Matt a lot between the different tests he was doing. He addressed us and Matt both, which not every doctor did. He had the CAT scan and proceeded to show us the tumor and the reason Matt's eyes were not reacting normally. The tumor was sitting on the optic nerve, which caused him to lose control of pupil dilation and the ability to look up on his own. He didn't duck with the bad news; he laid it on us. Matt had a tumor that could be malignant or not. If it was malignant it could be a germinoma or something else much worse. The germinoma was the most common brain tumor in children and was treatable with radiation and no operation. If it wasn't he would have to have heavy chemo and radiation and the tumor would have to be removed. This hung in the air for a moment as he exhaled even slower this time. But to determine that we must operate on Matt to relieve the pressure on his brain so the intense headache could be relieved and they could get a piece of tissue to do a biopsy. He explained the procedure to us, which sounded impossible to me, but he assured us that the risk was minimal.

Now I always had a knack of knowing how things worked but this just didn't make any sense to me. They would stick a needle in the top right portion of Matt's head and push the needle down to his tumor. There they would open up a place for the fluid to exit down his spine and relieve the pressure and at the same time try to pick off a bit of the tumor. The procedure would take less than an hour and Matt would feel better immediately. I wanted to understand how they did this without destroying other brain tissue, but like most other parents I just let the numbness take over and nodded my head.

On operation day I do not remember who watched our other children. It might have been my parents. It could have been Kathy's mother. It could have been anyone of ten or so people who helped us out every day. Again, we were lucky to have the support group we did. They were there for us every minute, every hour of every day. I often think of all the sick kids who didn't have that or how hard it is for kids whose parents didn't seem to care. Also, you wonder how hard it must be on single parents. I saw it all in the hospital, the very best and the very worst.

When we arrived it became a tradition that we got the residents first. They would come in and go through their checks and tests. They usually didn't talk to us except to say on departure that the doctor would be in. At first I thought this was a big waste of time and at times annoying, but as time went by I finally accepted their work as they needed to learn and Matt had some unique problems. His case was something different. Also, I'm sure it's a stress reliever for the doctor. He can't be on call 100 percent of the time.

As time went by Dr. Albright would do an exam, explaining the procedure to the resident as he went. In this case Matt had questions that were better than mine. He always listened even when you thought he wasn't paying attention. Dr. Albright, with his usual slow breathing and eyeing us up, told us what he was going to do, how long it would take, and what the outcome should be. He told us that this wasn't the best way to get tissue to biopsy but he needed to open a pathway to the spine to relieve pressure. At this point Dr. Albright asked us if we would pray with him. He prayed like he talked. I hoped God didn't get impatient with him. He was slow and deliberate with everybody. After the prayer nobody said anything. There was an uncomfortable silence until Dr. Albright started to talk about his life. He had been in the military and did his residency while in the service. He said he was very conflicted about becoming a doctor or a minister. I believed him. You could tell he still hadn't really made up his mind. He said the calling was strong but he thought the good he was doing with sick kids was good too.

Dr. Albright, you made the right choice. Maybe someday down the road you may change your career and there would be nothing wrong with that. I thank God every day you made the decision you did. You saved my son's life. Actually you have affected more lives and families then you will ever know. You pop into my mind for no reason sometimes. As dumb as it seems, I think it is the butterfly effect. As you help some other sick child, we all are with you to see your patient through. Maybe it's the only way I can do something for you.

The anesthesiologist took Matt and we would be able to see him when he awoke in recovery. The scary part was that Matt was way overdue. The social worker told us everything was okay and everybody acted differently to anesthetic. Dr. Albright eventually came out to see us and assured us everything had gone well. He wasn't sure about the tissue sample, but everything else was working properly. He said Matt should feel better immediately. When we saw him he had a wound that looked like the end of a nail file with an eyelet in the end. *[I still think it looks like I got kicked in the head by a horse.]* I still didn't see how they did it. Matt was fine as his headaches were gone. He was upbeat and was anxious to show his grandmother his new scar.

After surgery we decided to go on our family vacation, which was always Ocean City, MD. Kathy and I thought it would be good to get us a way for a few days and have some normalcy. We always go with my folks and my sister's family. They have two kids, Jill and Lauren, who are the same age, and our kids are close. I think it was a good idea. Even though there was the haze amongst us all, it was lifted a bit that week. There is comfort in family and friends. Kathy, Matt, and I headed back a few days early because we had a meeting with the radiologist. I do not have a great recollection of all that went on, but they had decided to use a gamma knife and Matt would have to get measured for the procedure. The gamma knife was like a football helmet on steroids. They would put it on Matt's head and there were hundreds of tiny sized, almost hair like, pathways that would focus radiation on the tumor, hence the measuring. It seemed to me it was newer technology as there seemed to be anxiety in the air as the radiologists talked more than they needed to. They were talking to each other and not us. It was going to be one shot of radiation and that would be it. They felt there would be less collateral damage. It was the first I heard this and I realized the complexity of what they were doing. Matt was thirteen. He was on the cusp of brain maturity. Radiation in younger children can cause permanent problems and a whole host of issues. Focusing all these beams to a single point would radiate tissue as it went through. When they intersected at the tumor that's where they would kill the cells. Mess up your math and a lot of bad things could happen. My mental state was turning a bit to the weary side. Keeping the adrenalin in check was difficult. My mind never stopped anymore it was on alert all the time.

When they were ready for us the first thing they did was take a new CT scan *[MRI]*. Then we went to take our turn to hurry up and wait. We waited longer than normal. I liked to walk around a lot and I was walking a marathon. Finally we went in and right away I knew we were in trouble. They were all there, the residents and the attendings. Someone nodded to the attending doctors and they started to explain. They were checking their measurements and something wasn't right. They discovered the tumor had grown considerably in the last week. They could not do the gamma knife procedure. They said that germinomas do not grow that fast. They were guessing it had to be another kind of cancer. I think all three of us wanted to cry but that would have been too good. I don't remember what they said after that because it didn't matter. We knew things were going to get worse. This was certainly a low point. It was the first time Matt seemed discouraged. We left and we were alone in our thoughts but we traveled together.

After a second biopsy, we were called back in and they had come to the conclusion that Matt had a malignant teratoma. They told us it was a very aggressive tumor and needed treatment right away. Dr. Albright and a Dr. Wollman were present, but Dr. Albright did all the talking. He said the tumor had to come out and that Matt would need heavy *chemo [he means chemotherapy]* and radiation. They said that chemo *[again he means chemotherapy]* was necessary because it was effective against aggressive tumors. Their eyes seemed to betray them. The ball game had changed. They had their game faces on. They didn't want to get too close anymore. We were entering a new phase of uncertainty. I felt cold. These guys deal with children's lives every day. They just can't get caught up in every emotional high and low. I changed that day. No more did I contemplate falling down, coming apart, or giving up. I would never give up. I now had purpose which gave me strength. I also found prayer that day.

Weird as it sounds, I had never prayed much. I didn't think it was right to pray for anything. I only prayed the normal prayers you say before bed. That ride home I prayed as hard as I could. I came up with a prayer that I memorized and repeated every day until present. I became a regular every morning at our Lady of Grace Parish in Greensburg. There is a prayer center in the church where I would kneel, and I was pretty much the only one there at 6:15 A.M. For some reason the doors were always open, so I thank the church leaders for that. There was a wooden Jesus a couple of feet tall that they have moved around a bit but which is always near the exit. When I got done with my prayer I would always high five him in a respectful way before I went out the door. Some of my best personal moments were in that church. I never told anybody before and I am not sure why I am now. It was the most intimate I have gotten with God and with myself. I believe prayer strengthened me.

We met with the doctors and they laid out the game plan for Matt's treatment. Again it was all business. He would have surgery immediately followed by chemo *[chemotherapy]* and then radiation. Dr. Albright would perform the surgery, Dr. Wollman would administer the chemo *[chemotherapy]* and Dr. Deutsch the radiation, in that order.

In looking back, the week before the operation all our friends and family got shoulder to shoulder and helped us through the week. The constant questions and wishes of good will were part of every conversation. There were times that I was patient and in control and other times I really didn't want to talk about it. Everybody handles things differently. I had my way. I tried not to convey a lot of emotion not that I didn't feel it but it would not have helped anything. I wanted to have a quiet confidence that would make everybody else comfortable. I know it was awkward for a lot of people to talk to me at all.

We got to the hospital early as Matt was to be one of the first cases in the OR that day. As Dr. Albright had explained earlier, he would make an incision from the base of his neck up about five inches. He would use a spatula to separate the brain and open a space to where he could get behind the eyes to remove the tumor. He said the operation could last four hours. When we got to pre op, we did the usual waiting but with a lot more anxiety. Nothing ever happened on time. Dr. Albright grabbed the three of us and went over what was going to happen one more time. After he finished he asked if it was all right if he prayed, and of course we nodded and he put together a short prayer that was direct and to the point. I think it calmed all of us. I know it calmed me.

Now was the hard waiting. I think it was the slowest time ever went for me. Minutes became hours and the hours seemed like days. About two hours into the operation the social worker came down and gave us an update. He said the operation was going smoothly but would take a while longer. He said the tumor was bloody so it was slow going, He said they removed the tumor using an instrument that would liquefy the tumor and then suction it out. It seemed out of place for him to talk details like that and I'm not sure we cared. We only heard it was proceeding smoothly. After four hours we saw the social worker again; the operation was over and Dr. Albright would be down momentarily to fill us in. As soon as I saw Dr. Albright I panicked. He had changed drastically in appearance. He was drawn and pale. His walk was heavy and he had a look that just screamed disaster. I spoke first and I was the one to panic. I said, "It didn't go very well did it?" He looked at me and said in a very loud and commanding voice, "No, quite the opposite. It could not have gone any better," and he meant it. I am one who reads a lot about the military and being in stressful situations. There are always stories about how pilots who would go out on long missions, be refueled in the air, and be in the cockpit for twelve hours. They said when the pilots were helped out of their planes they would look ten years older than when they left. After many months I realized that was the same thing here. The stress and the focus were so great that you would physically change your looks. I have to say I am embarrassed about this now. I wish I had let Dr. Albright speak first. He explained why it took so long and he said something peculiar. He only touched Matt once. I took that to mean he might have taken a few good cells with the bad, but he didn't dwell on it and neither did we.

They said we could see Matt in recovery after he woke up. Because of his other surgeries we knew he didn't react real well to anesthesia. Once we got the word we went to recovery and Matt was awake and talking. I was shocked and overcome by emotion. It appeared he made it through without any side effects. There was a giant exhale by everybody. I wondered how doctors get good at this stuff in the first place.

Matt was moved to the ICU after a couple of hours. I was shocked with every visit we made in there. I remember there were no windows in the place and there was a lot of stuff happening in there that was hard for me to grasp. I believe the unit held about twenty to twenty-five kids who ranged from infants to twenty year olds. Every kid in there was sicker than Matt. I wanted to cry every time I was there. It was the most uncomfortable I had been through the whole ordeal. There was a sixteen-year-old kid who fractured his vertebra and was paralyzed from the neck down. He was in a bed that flipped over every ten minutes to avoid bed sores. The infant next to Matt just had a liver transplant and the kid on the other side had just had open heart surgery. I gained a great deal of respect for the people that work there. It must be difficult and take a toll.

One quick story, and I wasn't there when it happened, but Matt, while still in the ICU, caused quite an uproar. When Kathy and I arrived to visit the nurse in charge came up to us visibly shaken but laughing at the same time. Apparently Matt had to pee real badly and he was supposed to tell the nurse so she could hold the bottle. I guess when you are thirteen the idea of a nurse holding your talywhacker is way more frightening than somehow making it to the bathroom. Apparently, when no one was watching, Matt got out of bed and found a stool (like a doctor would use) with wheels on it and shot himself across the unit to a bathroom. None of the nurses saw him until he tried to open the bathroom door. As you can imagine they were really shaken because he was not allowed up and if he had fallen it could have been disastrous. No harm no foul, but boy, were they buzzing like bees over that one.

The pathology report confirmed conclusively that it was a malignant teratoma. They said it was fairly rare. Apparently this type of tumor has cells like hair, nails, and other solid tissues in it. A few doctors said in passing that this might have been leftover cells of a twin. Matt's oncologist only remembered one other case that had this type of tumor in Pittsburgh. I never asked him what had happened. I didn't want to know.

Matt's recovery from surgery went really well. The surgery was successful and Matt was still the same person. We continued to see Dr. Albright monthly for checkups for a while, but his role in Matt's treatment became less and less. The person who was to become more influential and who we would soon formally meet was Dr. Wollman. We were told he was going to be Matt's oncologist and our go-to medical planner. The next step of treatment was going to be the most difficult. It seemed with this chemotherapy there were no guarantees that it would work. Chemotherapy was something that scared me. I always heard the word being associated with older people. It seemed to me to be a life extender but no cure. The side effects people complained of sounded worse than the disease. I thought it was a lot like bloodletting back in the Dark Ages, only this was by chemicals. I soon saw the kids with no hair and sad eyes looking a lot like Holocaust victims from WWII. Our son was going to be like that. I really tried to blank it out of my mind. Dr. Wollman, as we found out, was great at changing those expectations and made you feel better about the process. He had a way of telling you stuff straight but in a serene confident way.

On one fateful day we met with Dr. Albright's traveling residents and then with Dr. Albright himself. It seemed like on this day things were looking up as he talked much faster and with less ponderment. Maybe he was just getting to know us better. He led us over to oncology to formally meet Dr. Wollman. Dr. Wollman is as fine a human being that I ever met. We were lucky as Dr. Wollman and Matt clicked right away—enough humor to break the tension and a bedside manner that can only be described as a gift from God. Dr. Wollman talked to Kathy and me and always to Matt. Thirteen is a tough age, no longer just a kid but not yet a man. Dr. Wollman seemed to get it with Matt. In hindsight, I see how important this was for all of us. His relationship with Matt, and with my wife and myself, I can only describe as special. I often think of Dr. Wollman, and as strange as it seems I often think of his family. I know he is a great family man though I never met his family. To his wife and kids, I want to thank you for all those weekends and dinners he missed. For all the inconveniences you experienced and all the birthdays he got home late for. For all the days he came home tired and all the times when the stress was off the charts. For all the missed goodnight kisses. For all the extra work and planning your family had to do. For all the formal plastic smile functions that you had to attend. Most of all for all the love you had to share with all of us. Thank you is not justice, Dr. Wollman, but I know you get it.

The oncology team worked hard at putting together a combination of chemicals that would kill the cancer without killing Matt. It was not a refined science as not everybody reacted the same way to the drugs. Again, it was scary and I had no idea what to expect. They were throwing names around like cisplatin, carboplatin, and I can't remember what else. I used to have them all memorized and would look them up on the internet. That was quite stupid on my part as I did not understand one word. I appreciate the grueling hours these doctors put in to just keep up with what's new. It was around this time that Dr. Wollman also mentioned the tumor board. Apparently a group of doctors meet every week to review specific cancer cases and come up with treatments or, another word I learned, protocols. I always wanted to attend one of those meetings as I'm sure there was a lot of brain power in there with a healthy dose of ego. All the doctors that mentioned it seemingly looked forward to it. Maybe it's a sense of relief, all mechanics, no emotion, a let's-get-'er-done mentality. I would have liked to sit in on one of those meetings.

Dr. Wollman then went on to explain another concept. There were two, I'll call them groups, of hospitals that would share protocols and their effects on the patient. The two different groups would use these different protocols and then over time use the best one to treat their patients. I understand the idea and it makes a lot of sense to the medical community. As a father of a patient. I felt it was like playing a little bit of a betting game. Did I or did I not get the best most effective treatment? Maybe there was no answer, but it ignited the same feeling of helplessness in me anyway.

Dr. Wollman never did beat around the bush. Truth was always better, but hope was better yet. I eventually asked the question that most likely gets asked, and it was the only time I sensed a little bit of anger out of Dr. Wollman. I asked him, "What are Matt's chances?" The response was swift, practiced, and most importantly believed. "It doesn't matter what the chances are. Hope is there and that's all that matters." This turned out to be something I've taken with me for the rest of my life. There is a lot there when you think about it and a lot more when you practice it.

I am not a medical person, but when you get in these situations you either want to know more or you nod and turn off the short-term memory circuit. I went for the wanting to know more. Dr. Wollman was always patient and answered all the questions. He always had the right words and always told the truth. I had my concerns about Children's Hospital of Pittsburgh. Maybe it wasn't that great. I did a couple of things that were not out of desperation but with the idea that maybe, just maybe, I could have some influence over the whole situation. I started looking on the internet to see where we could go for a second opinion. I actually called Duke University School of Medicine and talked to the doctor in charge of Hematology/Oncology there. He was very interested in talking about Matt's case and showed a lot of interest in what the protocol was going to be for Matt. He told me that is not what they would have done. They would have changed the chemo [chemotherapy] drugs to something different. He was bordering on arrogant, but I respected the time he spent with me. If nothing else it caused me to look deeper into where we might go. The University of Pennsylvania had a great reputation at their Children's Hospital in Philadelphia. I called there and got buzzed around a lot but finally someone said yes, we could bring Matt over for a second opinion. We agreed on a date and went.

I'm not sure how Matt felt about this but I think he was a little bothered by it. He felt comfortable with the doctors he was already seeing and felt this was a waste of time. Even my wife I felt went along with it because I was talking it up so much. From where we live it was about a four-and-a-half hour drive to Philly. We got up real early as we had a mid-morning appointment. We were meeting with the head of oncology though I do not remember his name.   We got there and I remember it was a pretty nice facility, certainly newer than Pittsburgh's at that time. We checked in with the receptionist in the oncology clinic. She told us to take a seat and the doctor would be with us. Hurry up and wait turned into something completely different here. After about a three-hour wait and Matt and Kathy getting antsy, a doctor came out and introduced herself. She had a weird expression on her face and stumbled through her introduction. She apologized for the wait but there was some confusion. The doctor we were supposed to see had left the hospital for another job and nobody had gotten back to us. She said she had to see some of her patients but she would spend a little time with us. She realized we had come a long way and didn't want us to leave without getting what we came for. She asked for a rundown of Matt's treatment and how he was doing. She seemed like a real professional, and though you could tell she wanted or needed to go somewhere else she stayed and politely answered our questions. She did say she had one patient several years ago that had the same tumor as Matt. Their protocol was slightly different but she agreed with what they were doing in Pittsburgh. She also told us her patient was doing well after three years of being cancer free. She said the only side effect that she remembered was the girl had trouble with processing information but with work could learn and had the same IQ as before. She said, as a matter of fact, the girl wanted to get into medicine and the doctor thought she would do well.

After thanking her we picked up and headed down the PA turnpike. We talked for half an hour about the visit and laughed a little bit of how it was a waste of time and maybe Pittsburg was the right place for Matt. I also think Matt tucked the conversation in his subconscious. Maybe it wasn't a waste of time. The reason I bring this up is that we did tell Dr. Wollman about the second opinion and he said we did the right thing. As I said before, he always knew what to say. What a true professional.

In the end Matt had three chemo [chemotherapy] sessions. After each treatment he would wait three to four weeks before receiving the next one. The timing got pretty dependent on how he responded to the treatment. Matt's blood cells took a hit and he was getting blood tests all the time. Even when at home we often had to visit the local lab. The problem became more severe as Matt got further into the process. The focus became navigating that thin line between the positive and negative aspects of the chemo [chemotherapy]. This balancing act went on for about five months.

During those months we were often at the oncology clinic, where kids who were not in the hospital would be seen. It was located across the street from the hospital. This meant you had to go outside and walk a block or two to get there. As time went on you realized it was not a good situation. You still parked in the same stinky odorous garage and had to walk down the hill to Fifth Avenue and cross the street. If you needed to have preliminary tests in the hospital you then had to make this journey twice. As Matt's counts dropped it became difficult to walk that far. He would often have to stop and rest. The plus side was the office wasn't so hospital looking and had a bit of a warmer atmosphere. More importantly, the people who worked in the clinic were wonderful. First you would sign in and wait (nothing unusual there). Then they would draw Matt's blood and they had a machine on site that would print out all the pertinent facts about his blood and it did this in a short period of time. The doctors often waited until they got this information before they would see you. Dr. Wollman and Matt had a great relationship. The first five minutes of each encounter was a lot of one-up-manship and they would laugh, which was very important in my eyes. This five minutes was a gauge I believe they would use on each other to see where they were. As pressed for time as the doctors were, every one of them spent the right amount of time with you. We never felt like nobody cared.

It was a wonderful team and during this period the oncology department got a new head. They picked a great guy in Dr. Ritchey. When you are so focused as a parent and you like how things are going, this move was something my wife and I were worried about. He might come in and make big changes, which we didn't want to see happen. Dr. Ritchey proved not only that he knew what was going on but I think he made it better. He tried really hard to get the clinic back in the hospital. He was successful, but this was after our son's treatments had ended.

The nurses were terrific there too. Every time they saw you they were smiling. They were very genuine people who cared. They would help entertain siblings or sit with you a bit if the doctor was late. We seemed to get one nurse a lot named Donna. She had red hair and a great smile. She and Matt seemed to hit it off quite well. I want to thank her for always being so upbeat and personal. I believe she became pregnant right after Matt's treatments ended. I don't recall whether she had a boy or girl, but I'll bet she is a great mother.

Getting back to navigating that fine line, as the chemo *[chemotherapy]* continued Matt's counts bottomed out. This was a stressful period because Matt became much more susceptible to getting sick as his immune system became almost nonexistent. It was at this point Matt would have to often wear a mask to help him from picking up any bug. We tried hard to keep him away from other people, but that was harder than it sounds. There were always caring family, friends, and neighbors who wanted to see him. You could also tell that Matt would often get tired, but oddly enough he never complained. As we entered the final six weeks Matt would have to be admitted several times to the hospital for overnight stays because of fevers. Once they put him in isolation in that he had gotten that bad. During these episodes they would have to put Matt on an IV antibiotic. Matt was also on Dapsone chronically, for prophylactic reasons, which was normally used for people with leprosy.

One day after Dr. Wollman saw him, I remember him saying, "Matt, you are blue." It wasn't meant to be funny; he was blue. You could see Dr. Wollman's mind whirling. This was not something he dealt with every day. He was reaching for something he learned way back long ago but wasn't coming up with it. Some of the other doctors came over and were perplexed to. There were three of them. Finally Dr. Wollman said, "Matt you are being poisoned by the Dapsone." The other doctors laughed and kind of gave Dr. Wollman a professional pat on the back for coming up with that one. Fortunately for Matt they were able to change the antibiotic. Matt was no longer blue in a couple of days. In the end, Matt never got sick from the chemo itself. It was always the low blood counts that wore him down or some other impairment secondary from the treatment. It was a relief when it was all over. The constant monitoring and the clinic visits ran together and we may have had lost a fall season, but you might say it was the best we ever had.

During the chemo *[chemotherapy]*, it eventually came up. It started with his hair falling out a little at a time. Eventually it started to come out in chunks. We talked to Matt about maybe getting his head buzzed rather than going through all that mess. Eventually we got the go ahead from Matt and went to Fantastic Sam's and got it cut. They cut his hair in the back and didn't charge us, one of many random acts of kindness. He looked a lot different. The buzz look only lasted a few more days until the stubble fell out too. This is when you get that startling white appearance. I think Matt was embarrassed by this, but he never said anything. He had the look without the sad eyes. He could have made a commercial for Jerry Lewis's kids. Some of my friends shaved their heads to show him support.

Now that I am speaking about acts of kindness, a quick story. One of us always spent the night sleeping in the chair next to Matt's hospital bed. It was as uncomfortable as it looked. If I were a bigger person I wouldn't have been able to fit. Strangely, you figure out a few positions you can tolerate. Then again you have no choice. You were given a hospital blanket that was more kid sized and kind of fit like a postage stamp. I always slept in sweat pants and tee shirt. I think I burnt those clothes after all was said and done. Sleeping in the chair one night, curled up, a nurse woke me and wiped the drool off my chin. If this would have happened anywhere else I would have been embarrassed beyond belief. I made eye contact and thanked her. She smiled disarmingly and continued to make her rounds. It was a theme that got repeated over and over, simple acts of kindness.

When the chemo [chemotherapy] ended, Matt's blood counts began to rise, but we did have to wait a bit before they started the radiation process. In the meantime, they wanted to harvest stem cells from Matt. The procedure was quick and the cells were frozen in case he ever needed to have a bone marrow transplant. I don't remember how long they save the cells, so maybe somewhere in UPMC Matt's stem cells still sit. That whole concept was a little unnerving to me. It sort of popped out of nowhere. As the procedures moved on they were taking MRIs of Matt's head and spine to see if there was any more cancer. The reports were good, so we moved on.

Dr. Wollman told us the hospital was lucky to have the best radiation oncologist in the country and his name was Dr. Deutsch. I need to take a step back here: a radiation oncologist for kids, really? Before all this started I always thought that oncologists worked with the geriatric part of our population. Kids getting cancer and doctors specializing in treating pediatric cancer was something that didn't make sense. In my entire lifetime leading up to this I had never met a kid with cancer and the only thing I saw or heard were those St. Jude ads with Jerry Lewis. Now I was taking my son to see these people. Dr. Deutsch, I guess, was a big shot. Not only did he provide care for kids but for adults as well. As you walked into radiology, on the wall in the waiting room, there was a painting of Dr. Deutsch. It was a life-size replica done in oil, and as I remember it was almost like a photo. It was funny though. My guess is Dr. Deutsch had a patient he helped who wanted to thank him or his mother painted it at seventy-nine years young and he had no way out. I am glad he kept it there because it wasn't his ego; it was an act of kindness or love. I'm sure all the other doctors gave him a hard time!

When we met with Dr. Deutsch officially for the first time, he began with the potential effects that radiation could have on an immature brain. At thirteen Matt was a tweener, so he might experience some really bad side effects or none at all. As I asked my usual questions, this time I was blown away by how smart these guys have to be. Conversing with them, I got the impression that they would look at me and think, *You're not going to get it, so why ask?* but they always played along and humored me. I was overwhelmed again as I realized how helpless I was. It was not a simple process, quite the opposite. I also got the impression that you have to be a bit different to be a radiologist that does these kinds of treatments. I think the setup of how much radiation and where would take a lot of mathematics, and these guys appeared to have an interest in physics.

In the end Dr. Deutsch summarized the different options they had to treat Matt. Matt again always paid attention and asked good questions. Kathy was piecing it together and always strong. When the meeting was over the three of us were quiet as we made the journey home together. They were to call us when they got their game plan in order. I wish they had EZ Pass back then.

It seemed like it took them several weeks to get everything together, and Matt finally had to go to Presby to get a mask made up to fit his head. The mask was to hold his head still and to precisely position his head in the same position so the radiation would go where they wanted it with every treatment. The mask was eerie looking and wasn't something I liked to see. Once the mask was complete they started the treatments. They were going to radiate Matt's head and spine. I cannot recall why they treated the spine except that we were told it was a cancer that occurred in the centerline of the body. Later, when I was reading charts, apparently there was some disagreement whether there was something suspicious in two vertebrae of the spine. I never asked for an answer. They knew what they were doing. I was now a nodding father at this point.

Kathy ended up taking Matt down most of the times for his radiation treatments. The other kids were in school and I was at work. I think they had their little rituals and made the most of it. Outwardly the areas that were being radiated got red and dried out, but other than that Matt was good and he never complained. Debbie Ramsey, one of our neighbors, took Matt down for one of his treatments, taking all the neighborhood boys. Next door to us were the Stems, who had three boys, with Ted being the same age as Matt but going to a different school. The two younger boys were the same age as Zach and Jessie. The Ramsey's lived behind us and had three kids too. Their oldest was a girl, Erin, and then they had two boys, Justin and Ian, who were about the same age as our boys. The all grew up together and were close. Debbie, on the way home, stopped at the local Hooters. It was a memorable day for them and another act of kindness that helped along the way.

It took six weeks, but Matt was finished. I have to tell you, that was another weird time for me. *Finished* meant that Matt would not be getting looked at darn near every day, which was our safety blanket and was going to come to an end. You almost wanted to go in and beg them to keep seeing him every week. I was helpless, and now we were in a new stage where there wasn't help anymore at all.

My mind would get into the *what ifs*, but I tried to think the opposite, that it would be great to get back to normal. The *what ifs* still come around today, but not as often. Will that ever go away? I don't think so.

While the treatments ended, our follow up visits and MRIs continued. The five days leading up to the scan was really nerve-wracking. I don't think any of us talked about it. We would see what we would see. I was the designated person to take Matt to these. They would let me sit in the room with him as long as I emptied my pockets of metal. It took about an hour to run one of the scans. It never seemed to bother Matt going into the cylindrical tube where the machine would do its thing. Sitting in there I always prayed a lot and tried to figure out what all the different noises it made were from. I pretty much had the pattern down by the end. Sometimes I thought they were fake and they just added those sounds to keep your mind occupied.

Most of the time we had the same technician and her name was Patty. Again, she was terrific in getting everything set up and giving Matt his contrast. She always asked him if he was all right, and Matt would always be okay except once. At the halfway point of the scan they inject you with contrast to give you a more accurate picture. On this day she said they were using a new brand. She put it in his IV and he got in the machine, and within a minute Matt said he needed out and he was going to be sick. As soon as he sat up he barfed over everything. It was the most violent sick I ever saw him. Patty put it in his chart to use the good stuff from then on. Matt and I would go every month for eighteen months and then once a quarter and then once a year. Every trip produced a high level of anxiety until the clinic called back with results. Waiting for the results would take some time off your life. If they missed their promised time you would call immediately. All the people were pleasant and understood your concern, but going over the limit was excruciatingly painful. Every parent going through this I'm sure can tell you how soul searchingly hard it was. Ten years after being treated Matt had his last MRI.

To the Parents

I'm sure that I was no different than other parents before this happened. You never grow up and figure you will be in such a helpless position. As a parent you are in charge and have 100 percent responsibility to see your child to adulthood. As a parent of a sick child you fixate on asking yourself how you could have let this happen. You pray to God to give you the cancer. You complain that it is not fair. I feel I need to give some perspective on being a parent of a sick kid. As I said before, you feel helpless, which stems from the feeling that you know nothing, *zip*. It is a difficult time, maybe the most difficult. I lapsed into this train of thought on and off again, but remember, you can't possibly understand everything and do everything.

Feeling sorry for yourself can feel pretty good, and when that happened to me I got a dose of reality that made me thankful for everything I had. One night we were in the hospital room with one other child. All the other rooms were taken, so you did the best you could, but nobody really cared as we were all in the same predicament. We all had kids getting treated for cancer, so privacy or personal interests just didn't matter. As it got later in the evening, after numerous walks around the floor, numerous visitations, numerous games being played, and just meaningless chatter to chew up time, it was time to get ready for bed. Matt got in his bed and I was sitting in my chair, soon to be my bed, when the mother of the child next to us was putting on her PJs, and the last thing she did was take off her wig. She had her head down a bit sheepishly, and I asked her if she was being treated for cancer too. She nodded and said she was into her sixth month of treatment. I was so dumb struck by the idea that she was enduring cancer while her child was being treated too, and I was at a loss for any words to say. I knew from talking to them before she was a single mother. Her child was four or five years old and she was going through this alone. The next day when I saw my wife I hugged her and told her the story. Even writing this today, seventeen years later, I cried. Her child passed away several months later and I never heard how things went with her.

When Matt had cancer I worked for Menasha Corporation and we had a customer I handled called Haskell. They made office furniture. They had a guy who worked there, and as it turned out he had a son treated at Children's Hospital for leukemia. We ended up meeting several times and we talked at great lengths about Children's Hospital and the work they did. He knew the doctors. He knew the nurses and was a beacon of light for me. He was giving me grounding for what we were going to go through. I found out from somebody else that his son had died at eighteen, which he never told me at first. When I saw him again I brought it up and he went through the whole story. He said his son was never discouraged and always up-beat except for the last couple of months. I felt him bearing his soul though he still had that wall up. He was still in that fog, but he couldn't have been more glowing about the care his son got. One day he stopped me and said he really had something that was important to tell me. He said, "Look, the most important thing you have to be aware of is the statistic that couples with really sick kids or kids that have passed, they have a divorce rate over 75 percent." He hesitated and looked me square in the eye and said, "You will blame each other for the health problems of your son or daughter without question. Unless you or your wife keeps that out front in your marriage, it will happen to you." Silence. I never had or have had anybody tell me something with more conviction and emotion than what was just said to me. As the years have rolled by I can see how it could happen. Funny how people you aren't necessarily that close with can have that kind of impact. I hope he learned the same. I looked his stats up and it was 77 percent. I hope every family who goes through this gets that advice. *It is not your or anyone else's fault. Never forget it.*

To Caregivers

I have a very profound vision of what our caregivers go through on a daily basis. It's love, it's heartache, it's purposeful, it's stressful, it's rewarding, it's thankless, it's professional, it's exhausting, and it has great meaning, but sometimes it seems all for naught when things don't go the right way. All the caregivers at the hospital who helped us through all of Matt's cancer, I cannot thank enough. Writing this has caused me to really see and appreciate what you do every day. Our family has been blessed with a lot of people in medicine. My wife is a nurse, my sister is a nurse, my mother is a nurse, my mother-in-law was a nurse, my father-in-law was a doctor, and now my two sons are doctors and my youngest daughter is on her way to being a physician's assistant. They all have ups and downs about what they are doing, but they all care and have worked hard to be the best they can be. I hope they all practice medicine with the same care we received at Children's Hospital of Pittsburgh. If you ever have a sick kid who needs extra care, Children's Hospital of Pittsburgh is a fantastic place. The amount of brain power there is off the charts. We did not work with anybody who was not supportive or who didn't have enough time. To the nurses, social workers, aides, cleaning people, administrators, doctors and everybody who we came in contact with I give you a belated thank you. Though there are times when you forget and don't see it, you are all members of a very important team. You save children's lives. Nobody can give this kind of care by themselves so take one moment to acknowledge the person next to you and appreciate what can be right about medicine. My wife and I cannot thank you enough.

Family, Friends, and Supporters

There was a lot of other stuff going around at this time too, and Matt and I need to speak to those who supported with these matters. The doctors told us we had to pull him out of school. He would be home taught for the whole school year. Greater Latrobe School District did a great job in sending teachers to do the home schooling. *[Their names were Dr. Rullo and Mrs. Agostinone.]* Each would spend a half a day every week with Matt covering all the required seventh grade materials. They were terrific. Kathy and Matt obviously became pretty close with them. I was outside the loop most of the time at work and did not have a lot of interaction. They were professional and they never seemed like it was a pain in the butt.

As mentioned before, I worked at Menasha Corporation's Yukon Plant at the time Matt was sick. A couple of days before Matt's operation I went to work to meet with our management team. I was the general manager and I knew, with all that was going on, my time would be limited at work. Word had already spread about what had happened so there was an unusual quietness as I made my way to my office. I was really nervous as I wasn't sure I was going to be able to talk about the situation without going to pieces. I remember I had everybody come into my office, and as they assembled I could tell they were as nervous as me. I was blessed to have a group I could rely on as much as these people. Thank you John Fullerton, Tom Huber, Bob Yutz, Carrie Boord, Jim Roberts, and all the people of Menasha Corporation's Yukon plant. Everybody picked up the ball—or maybe I should say picked me up and we moved forward together. I know everybody prayed for Matt; it made a difference. I will never forget this love and support. This will last forever. I made it through the explanation of what was happening only because they were great people. On the way home that day I cried a little, one of the few times I got that pleasure.

I also need to thank our neighbors. Christmas that year was made extra special because of them. Twelve days from Christmas we anonymously received a partridge in a pear tree. The next day came two turtle doves, then came three French hens, and so on. On the morning of Christmas Eve they were all singing the Twelve Days of Christmas in our front yard. Thank you for all the well wishes, even from people I had never met but who had heard about Matt; it all helped.

Now to all Kathy's and my brothers and sisters who chipped in and made things more tolerable and to our nieces and nephews who encouraged Matt and accepted him at face value: Nobody ever lost faith and all realized something different was going on here. They hoped beyond hope that Matt would do well. I want to especially thank Kathy's brother, Bobby *[Father Jude Peters]*, who had people all over the world praying for Matt in his recovery. I also need to especially thank my sister, Char, for the time she spent with our other children during this time in our lives. She tried to make their life a little special as well. Finally, to my mother-in-law, Jean, and my mother and father, Chuck and Bert, I thank you for watching our kids all the numerous times we had to be in Pittsburgh with Matt. Thank you for helping out with meals, for helping with school work, for being there to get them to bed and to get them to the bus, and for taking them places to occupy their time when we could not. Matt knew your unconditional love was a big part of his recovery. I thank you for all your patience and strength you showed through this experience. It helped me stay grounded and gave me hope and an inner faith that everything would be okay.

I don't know how to describe what our other kids went through. They had many questions and they had many feelings that I did not know how to deal with. It was hard for them to understand the intensity level Kathy and I were at. We got very focused on Matt and the whole healing process. Even 17 years later when writing these words I can feel that fog closing back in smothering all emotions. They all have said they wished we would have told them more. I don't know if I could have. As I said before if the damn broke you sure as heck didn't want it to happen in front of them. Maybe I was protecting myself more than them. I want to come up with more words to talk about them and this period of our lives but it isn't there. I don't really remember. To Zach, Jess and Cait please forgive me. Every waking minute was spent trying to figure out how to get rid of

Matt's cancer and getting him the care he needed. All else went on hold. Time stood still for a year. I will say Matt could not have a better supporting brother and sisters than you. Till this day you have stood by him through thick and thin. You have made me proud and content in my role. If I had a magic wand I would make all childhood illnesses go away. As our kids have grown older I think they have begun to realize what this lost year was all about. I hope they see more clearly how fragile and how unpredictable life can be.

Finally I want to thank my wife. I want to thank her for all the talks, all the strength, and all the love she put into everything. I don't know how a single parent could cope with all this without having someone to lean on or confide in. Kathy did so much to keep our family's lives as normal as possible through Matt's treatments and recovery. My wife, thankfully, is the most organized person on the planet. I never remember ever setting up who was going to watch the kids, who was going to get dinner, who was going to stay in Pittsburgh, or who was packing whose bag. She did all that twenty-four hours a day. I worked as much as I could and she did the rest. She was our rock, and I can't thank her enough for her love and positive outlook. I realize even more now how important this was in getting Matt better and keeping me on an even keel. We took turns staying with Matt at the hospital, but it was Kathy who kept the home front running. We did talk about the advice we got and I think it was really good. Going through an experience like this will point out all the flaws in your relationship or make you both appreciate what you have even more. I like to think it was growth for the both of us. We really don't talk about it much anymore, but there are things that trigger your emotions and I know we can look at each other and know what the other is thinking. Thank you, Kathy, for being the best wife and mother you possibly could. I wouldn't have made it through this experience intact without you.

Matt

I really didn't talk a lot about Matt the person. I wrote this from a parent's perspective, thinking that it might help some other mother or father who is going through the same thing. Matt was thirteen when he got cancer, and for a year he pretty much never had a normal moment. Matt gained a lot and lost some because of cancer, but when looking back I never remember him complaining. He was pretty quiet, though he had a very good idea of what was going on. Matt did question a lot of things to get an understanding and knew more about what was going on than you could take at face value. He had a great relationship with his doctors and it was good for him. He would always spar with Dr. Wollman before getting down to business. Actually, I think Dr. Wollman used it to gauge where Matt was mentally, emotionally, and physically. The nurses and technical people were important to Matt as well. I always thought those acts of kindness he received from these caregivers went a long way for Matt. In return he was always kind and respectful. I think he realized the job they all had to do.

Physically, Matt never grew anymore once he had cancer. He stayed about the same size—not that he was going to be a giant, but his build has remained the same since he was diagnosed. He lost his pituitary gland to the radiation and he has no growth hormone. He ended up going through a lot of testing with an endocrinologist to get some of his hormones back to where they needed to be, but even today he has to take daily shots to his stomach to keep his system in balance. It's an everyday reminder of something from the past. Socially, Matt also experienced some hardships. At home Matt's relationship changed with the other kids as he was getting all the attention. He sometimes felt the wrath of his brother and sisters. Unfortunately, Matt kind of shut them out for a while. Rather than find out what they were up to or spend time with them, he just kind of ignored them. During his treatment his grandparents became his go-to people. I think he felt they would accept him as is and cancer be damned. His relationship with them continues to this day. Junior high is a big time with regard to social development, and I think Matt missing that year hurt him in his social development later in life. Academically though he did very well and passed. I think there is way more here than what I am briefly mentioning, but truly it was a big deal.

I think for Matt humor played a big part in getting over this experience. When he was hospitalized, rather than dwelling on all the negatives, I think Matt used humor to keep things in perspective. I also think it got him better. It mentally helped in beating back the negative emotions associated with the disease. I may be wrong about this, but I think Matt grew with God as well. I know it changed my relationship with God. Matt often talked of being a priest but he always wanted to be a doctor. Even before cancer he talked of it. In reality, I really wonder how Matt felt inside. The truth is, I never asked him. I don't know why that was but I felt it seemed too intrusive to ask him to pour out his inner most thoughts. I'm not sure I wanted to know either. Writing about his story has really helped me see and understand what he was thinking and what he as a person went through. Maybe this will help us both get to the next chapter.

Matt was not the most outgoing kid before cancer, but he had friends and never thought twice about going out to play, but after cancer he did not seem as interested in making relationships and became more introspective. I have often thought that having to deal with a real life-and-death situation placed him in a world that others wouldn't understand. I do feel closeness with Matt that comes with going through this kind of experience. Sometimes I hang on every word he says. He's the only person who I ask "How you are doing?" and wait anxiously for a response. It never goes away.

Matt became very focused on becoming a doctor. I do believe that his cancer experience taught him to have an inner tenacity that got him through some rough times. Many times he could have folded the tent as studying the hours it took him to get through med school consumed his every waking moment. I've often thought about the doctor in Philly who talked about not losing IQ but your brain doesn't process information as quickly. I kind of think that about Matt. Nobody can ever take that from him, and he got that through this cancer experience. I am happy to report that Matt graduated from med school in 2010. He is currently a resident at UPMC in family medicine. I am very proud of his accomplishments and admire his ability to persevere and overcome adversity. Matt, I love you and you have done well. May this experience help us all in being better people, and maybe sharing this story can give a child or parent a bit of hope or ray of sunshine in their lives while they go through this up and down journey.

When Matt was sick they always played the song "I Believe I Can Fly" on the radio while driving to and from the hospital, so every time I hear it takes me back. Matt, you are the best. I can't wait to read your story!